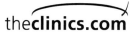

ORTHOPEDIC CLINICS
OF NORTH AMERICA

Oncology

GUEST EDITOR
Rakesh Donthineni, MD

January 2006 • Volume 37 • Number 1

SAUNDERS

An Imprint of Elsevier, Inc.
PHILADELPHIA   LONDON   TORONTO   MONTREAL   SYDNEY   TOKYO

W.B. SAUNDERS COMPANY
A Division of Elsevier Inc.

Elsevier Inc., 1600 John F. Kennedy Blvd., Suite 1800, Philadelphia, PA 19103-2899.

http://www.orthopedic.theclinics.com

ORTHOPEDIC CLINICS OF NORTH AMERICA
January 2006
Editor: Debora Dellapena

Volume 37, Number 1
ISSN 0030-5898
ISBN 1-4160-3383-1

The ideas and opinions expressed in *Orthopedic Clinics of North America* do not necessarily reflect those of the Publisher. The Publisher does not assume any responsibility for any injury and/or damage to persons or property arising out of or related to any use of the material contained in this periodical. The reader is advised to check the appropriate medical literature and the product information currently provided by the manufacturer of each drug to be administered to verify the dosage, the method and duration of administration, or contraindications. It is the responsibility of the treating physician or other health care professional, relying on independent experience and knowledge of the patient, to determine drug dosages and the best treatment for the patient. Mention of any product in this issue should not be construed as endorsement by the contributors, editors, or the Publisher of the product or manufacturers' claims.

Orthopedic Clinics of North America (ISSN 0030-5898) is published quarterly (For Post Office use only: Volume 37 issue 1 of 4) by Elsevier Inc. Corporate and editorial offices: Elsevier Inc., 1600 John F. Kennedy Blvd., Suite 1800, Philadelphia, PA 19103-2899. Accounting and circulation offices: 6277 Sea Harbor Drive, Orlando, FL 33887-4800. Periodicals postage paid at Orlando, FL 32862, and additional mailing offices. Subscription prices are $190.00 per year for (US individuals), $315.00 per year for (US institutions), $225.00 per year (Canadian individuals), $370.00 per year (Canadian institutions), $260.00 per year (international individuals), $370.00 per year (international institutions), $95.00 per year (US students), $130.00 per year (Canadian and international students). Foreign air speed delivery is included in all *Clinics* subscription prices. All prices are subject to change without notice. POSTMASTER: Send address changes to *Orthopedic Clinics of North America*, W.B. Saunders Company, Periodicals Fulfillment, Orlando, FL 32887-4800. **Customer Service: 1-800-654-2452 (US). From outside of the US, call 1-407-345-4000. E-mail: hhspcs@harcourt.com.**

Reprints. For copies of 100 or more, of articles in this publication, please contact the Commercial Reprints Department, Elsevier Inc., 360 Park Avenue South, New York, New York 10010-1710. Tel. (212) 633-3813 Fax: (212) 462-1935 e-mail: reprints@elsevier.com

Orthopedic Clinics of North America is covered in *Index Medicus, Cinahl, Excerpta Medica,* and *Cumulative Index to Nursing and Allied Health Literature.*

Printed in the United States of America.

GUEST EDITOR

RAKESH DONTHINENI, MD, Assistant Professor, Department of Orthopedic Oncology, University of California, Davis Medical Center, Sacramento, California

CONTRIBUTORS

ADESEGUN ABUDU, FRCS, Royal Orthopaedic Hospital, Birmingham, United Kingdom

ANDREAS ADAM, FRCP, FRCS, FRCR, Professor of Interventional Radiology, Department of Radiology, Guy's and St. Thomas' Hospital, London, United Kingdom

LUIS A. APONTE-TINAO, MD, Orthopaedic Oncology Service, Institute of Orthopedics Carlos E. Ottolenghi, Italian Hospital of Buenos Aires, Buenos Aires, Argentina

MIGUEL A. AYERZA, MD, Orthopaedic Oncology Service, Institute of Orthopedics Carlos E. Ottolenghi, Italian Hospital of Buenos Aires, Buenos Aires, Argentina

SIMON CARTER, FRCS, Royal Orthopaedic Hospital, Bristol Road South, Birmingham, United Kingdom

THOMAS DELANEY, MD, Associate Professor, Harvard Medical School; Department of Medical Oncology, Massachusetts General Hospital, Boston, Massachusetts

RAKESH DONTHINENI, MD, Assistant Professor, Department of Orthopedic Oncology, University of California, Davis Medical Center, Sacramento, California

JEFFERY J. ECKARDT, MD, Professor, Division of Orthopedic Oncology, University of California Los Angeles, Los Angeles, California

FREDERICK R. EILBER, MD, Professor, Division of Surgical Oncology, University of California Los Angeles, Los Angeles, California

FRITZ C. EILBER, MD, Assistant Professor, Division of Surgical Oncology, University of California Los Angeles, Los Angeles, California

EDWARD J. FOX, MD, Assistant Professor, Department of Orthopedic Oncology, University of Pennsylvania, Philadelphia, Pennsylvania

AFSHIN GANGI, MD, PhD, Professor of Radiology, University Louis Pasteur, University Hospital of Strasbourg, Strasbourg, France; Honorary Consultant Interventional Radiologist, Guy's and St. Thomas' Hospital, London, United Kingdom

ROBERT GRIMER, FRCS, Royal Orthopaedic Hospital, Birmingham, United Kingdom

JAMES B. HAYDEN, MD, PhD, Department of Orthopedics and Rehabilitation, Oregon Health and Science University, Portland, Oregon

BANG H. HOANG, MD, Department of Orthopaedic Surgery, Chao Family Comprehensive Cancer Center, University of California, Irvine, California

HARISH S. HOSALKAR, MD, MBMS, FCPS, Diplomate, National Board of Orthopaedic Surgeons; Department of Orthopedic Oncology, University of Pennsylvania, Philadelphia, Pennsylvania

RONALD HUGATE, Jr, MD, Colorado Limb Consultants, Denver, Colorado

SAFDAR N. KHAN, MD, Resident, Department of Orthopaedic Surgery, University of California at Davis Medical Center, Sacramento, California

RICHARD D. LACKMAN, MD, Chairman of Orthopaedic Surgery, Department of Orthopedic Oncology, University of Pennsylvania, Philadelphia, Pennsylvania

D. LUIS MUSCOLO, MD, Professor of Orthopaedics, Chairman, Institute of Orthopedics Carlos E. Ottolenghi, Italian Hospital of Buenos Aires, Buenos Aires, Argentina

SCOTT D. NELSON, MD, Associate Professor, Division of Pathology, University of California Los Angeles, Los Angeles, California

ONDER OFLUOGLU, MD, Vice Chair, Orthopedic Surgery and Trauma Clinic, Lutfi Kirdar Education and Research Hospital, Istanbul, Turkey

CHRISTIAN M. OGILVIE, MD, Orthopaedic Resident, Department of Orthopedic Oncology, University of Pennsylvania, Philadelphia, Pennsylvania

TARUN SABHARWAL, FRCSI, FRCR, Consultant Interventional Radiologist, Department of Radiology, Guy's and St. Thomas' Hospital, London, United Kingdom

RICHARD SALTER, MRCS, FRCR, Interventional Radiology Fellow, Department of Radiology, Guy's and St. Thomas' Hospital, London, United Kingdom

FRANKLIN H. SIM, MD, Department of Orthopedic Surgery, Division of Orthopedic Oncology, Mayo Clinic, Rochester, Minnesota

WILLIAM D. TAP, MD, Fellow, Division of Medical Oncology, University of California Los Angeles, Los Angeles, California

RICHARD M. TEREK, MD, Associate Professor, Department of Orthopaedic Surgery, Brown University, Providence, Rhode Island

ROGER TILLMAN, FRCS, Royal Orthopaedic Hospital, Birmingham, United Kingdom

JESSE T. TORBERT, MD, Department of Orthopedic Oncology, University of Pennsylvania, Philadelphia, Pennsylvania

ROBERT E. TURCOTTE, MD, FRCSC, Associate Professor and Chairman, Division of Orthopaedic Surgery, McGill University; Director, Department of Orthopaedic Surgery, McGill University Health Centre, Montreal, Quebec, Canada

CONTENTS

FORTHCOMING ISSUES

RECENT ISSUES

VISIT THESE RELATED WEB SITES

Access your subscription at:
www.theclinics.com

ELSEVIER
SAUNDERS

Orthop Clin N Am 37 (2006) ix

ORTHOPEDIC
CLINICS
OF NORTH AMERICA

Preface

Oncology

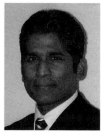

Rakesh Donthineni, MD
Guest Editor

We have come a long way, from the concept of the four humors in the body as described by Hippocrates and the dogmas of Galen to the improvement in sterility that resulted from Lister's discoveries in the nineteenth century. The advances have been even more dramatic within the last century. As we progress through the technological revolution, medicine has kept in step, making possible rapid changes and affecting the way physicians practice. With regard to musculoskeletal tumor management, the last 3 decades have taken us from a time of treatment primarily by amputation, with survival for sarcomas still poor, to an era of limb-sparing surgeries and the impact of chemotherapies on overall survival. Newer techniques have significantly affected patient care; these include diagnostics using cell and molecular tests, cytogenetics, radiologic tests, better drugs to treat the cancers, and improved, longer-lasting reconstruction material that allows soft tissue attachments. The quality of research on bone and soft tissue tumors is evident in the number of presentations at the national and international meetings dedicated to our specialty. This edition of the *Orthopedic Clinics of North America*, dedicated to orthopedic oncology, reviews some of the latest concepts in basic science and clinical medicine affecting the field.

I am grateful to the authors from various parts of the world for their contributions and dedication to this specialized area of orthopedics. Much gratitude also to Deb Dellapena, the editor at Elsevier, for coordinating the chapters and making this a successful endeavor.

Rakesh Donthineni, MD
Department of Orthopedic Oncology
University of California, Davis Medical Center
4860 Y Street, Suite 3800
Sacramento, CA 95817, USA
E-mail address: rakesh.donthineni@ucdmc.ucdavis.edu

ELSEVIER
SAUNDERS

Orthop Clin N Am 37 (2006) 1 – 7

ORTHOPEDIC
CLINICS
OF NORTH AMERICA

Osteosarcoma: Basic Science and Clinical Implications

James B. Hayden, MD, PhD[a], Bang H. Hoang, MD[b],*

[a]Department of Orthopedics and Rehabilitation, Oregon Health & Science University, 3181 SW Sam Jackson Park Road,
OP 31, Portland, OR 97239, USA
[b]Department of Orthopaedic Surgery, 101 The City Drive, University of California, Irvine Medical Center, Orange,
CA 92868, USA

Osteosarcoma is a primary malignancy of bone with a high tendency to metastasize. Although it can occur at any age, osteosarcoma has a peak incidence in the second decade with a second peak of incidence in the elderly population. The most common locations in young patients are areas with rapid bone growth, such as the distal femur, proximal tibia, and proximal humerus [1]. Common locations in older adults are more axial and occur in areas that have been previously irradiated or have underlying bone abnormalities such as Paget's disease.

Current treatment recommendations for osteosarcoma include neoadjuvant chemotherapy and surgical resection, followed by postoperative chemotherapy. Chemotherapy protocols involve multiagents and may include doxorubicin, cisplatin, ifosfamide, and methotrexate [2]. Surgical resection requires a wide margin, and limb salvage has become the standard with little change in the local recurrence rate [2]. Prognostic indicators for osteosarcoma include metastatic disease; size and location of the tumor; response to neoadjuvant chemotherapy; and surgical remission [1,3]. Response to chemotherapy is measured as the percent of histologic necrosis in the resected specimens, with a good response being more than 90% necrosis [3].

Osteosarcoma can be divided into several subtypes. Conventional osteoblastic osteosarcoma makes up approximately 70% of all osteosarcomas. Chondroblastic and fibroblastic osteosarcomas are the next most common at approximately 10% each. Less common types of osteosarcoma include anaplastic, telangiectatic, giant-cell rich, and small cell [3]. The response to chemotherapy is best with fibroblastic subtypes and poorest with the chondroblastic subtypes [3].

Of patients who present with no metastatic disease, approximately 70% will be long-term survivors. The remaining patients will develop a relapse. The average time to relapse is 1.6 years and 95% of the relapses will occur within the first 5 years [4]. Pulmonary metastasis is the most common form of distant spread (in 80% of patients), with bone involvement being the second most common mode of spread (in 15% of patients) [4]. The average survival after a recurrence is less than 1 year. Of those who do achieve a second remission, 70% to 80% will develop a second relapse within 1 year [4].

When a poor responder is identified, attempts are made to intensify the therapy. This therapeutic intensification is often accomplished by changing chemotherapy agents or by increasing the dosage with a few protocols trying stem cell rescue. Unfortunately, this procedure has not been demonstrated to increase long-term survival [5]. However, in patients who develop a surgically resectable recurrence or metastasis, resection has been shown to improve survival.

Research in osteosarcoma has been focused on identifying which patients will respond to the current therapy. The goal is to identify the patients whose tumor will resist chemotherapy or whose tumor will metastasize or recur. These patients could potentially

---

* Corresponding author.
E-mail address: bhhoang@uci.edu (B.H. Hoang).

doi:10.1016/j.ocl.2005.06.004

orthopedic.theclinics.com

be treated differently. The second area of focus has been to identify new targets for therapy that may be more effective or less toxic, especially for the tumors that respond poorly to the conventional agents.

Etiology

Understanding the etiology of osteosarcoma may provide some clues for therapeutic strategy. Unfortunately, most osteosarcoma cases are random, with few known environmental exposures or genetic associations [6,7]. There are a few diseases that are known to increase the risk for osteosarcoma. Patients who have retinoblastoma have a mutation in the Rb tumor suppressor gene, resulting in a significantly higher risk for developing osteosarcoma and other malignancies. Li-Fraumeni syndrome involves a mutation in the p53 tumor suppressor gene. These patients are at increased risk for multiple malignancies, including osteosarcoma. Rb and p53 are involved in cell cycle regulation [8]. Mutations in p53 have been found consistently in osteosarcoma; however, its role in advanced disease is controversial [9,10].

Other syndromes associated with osteosarcoma include Rothmund-Thomson syndrome and Bloom syndrome. Rothmund-Thomson syndrome is associated with a mutation in the RECQL4 gene and Bloom syndrome is caused by a mutation in the BLM gene [8]. These genes are DNA helicases, enzymes that help unwind the DNA to allow duplication.

There are few known environmental exposures that cause osteosarcoma. The only chemical exposure known includes beryllium oxide, which has been shown to cause osteosarcoma in an animal model [8]. The virus FBJ has been shown to induce osteosarcoma in mice, but no known infectious agent has been shown to cause osteosarcoma in humans [8]. Up to 50% of osteosarcomas demonstrate SV40 viral DNA [11]. The significance of this finding is unknown.

Radiation therapy has been associated with the development of secondary osteosarcoma. The dose of radiation required for this is not known, but is probably significantly above that encountered for regular diagnostic procedures. Radiation-induced osteosarcoma risk is increased with increasing dose of radiation and a younger age at exposure. Another cause of secondary osteosarcoma is a primary bone abnormality. The most common of these is Paget's disease, with approximately 1% of patients who have Paget's disease developing osteosarcomas.

Chromosomal abnormalities

Chromosomal abnormalities are common in osteosarcomas. Approximately 70% of osteosarcomas will show some chromosomal abnormality, including gains and losses. Consistently identified abnormalities include a gain of chromosome 1; loss of chromosomes 9, 13, and 17; partial loss of chromosome 6q; and rearrangements involving chromosomes of 11, 19, and 20 [11]. Some of these abnormalities are consistent with the syndromes that are associated with osteosarcoma. For instance, the Rb gene for retinoblastoma maps to chromosome 13q and p53 for Li-Fraumeni maps to 17p. Loss of these chromosomal regions could create defects similar to those in patients who have the genetic mutations.

In normal cells, shortening of telomeres at the ends of chromosomes is responsible for senescence. Tumor cells escape normal senescence by aberrantly maintaining telomere length. There are two mechanisms to maintain telomere length as the chromosome duplicates. The first uses a telomerase, which lengthens the telomere, and the second is a recombination-based method using the alternative lengthening of telomere (ALT) pathway. About 50% of osteosarcomas are dependent on the ALT pathway to evade senescence [11]. The ALT pathway is associated with more chromosomal instability, which may explain the large variations of chromosomal defects associated with osteosarcoma. In an animal model, a telomerase pathway was associated more closely with metastatic potential [11]. Therefore, the telomere maintenance mechanisms may function as an early marker for more aggressive disease.

DNA microarray

DNA microarray analysis is a technique that allows analysis of the expression of multiple genes to be completed simultaneously. This powerful new technique is being applied to osteosarcomas. The analysis is usually completed in two ways. The first is to identify clusters of genes that may be prognostic as a group. Prognostic clusters may identify genes that are increased or decreased in their expression level in metastatic versus nonmetastatic or in chemotherapy-sensitive versus -nonsensitive tumors. The second method is to identify cellular signaling pathways that provide insight into the etiology or may be targets for novel therapy.

Microarray analysis has been used in an attempt to identify patients who will respond poorly to the chemotherapy. A cluster analysis comparing patients who have poor chemotherapy response with patients who have good response identified 104 genes that were found to be statistically different. The group that had a poor response to chemotherapy was noted to have expression changes in pathways that stimulated osteoclast development and activity, extracellular matrix remodeling, and apoptosis resistance [12]. Another group of investigators used microarray to analyze six responders and seven nonresponders. The investigators identified 60 genes and were able to separate the two groups. Prominent among these were genes thought to be involved in chemotherapy resistance, such as AKR1C4, GPX1, and GSTTLp28 [13]. Other investigators have used microarray to evaluated differences in gene expression before and after chemotherapy. This comparison demonstrated an increased expression of DNA repair genes [14].

Microarray analysis has also been used to identify the characteristics of tumors more likely to be metastatic. Human cell lines with high and low metastatic potential were identified and subjected to microarray analysis. There was differential expression of seven genes in the metastatic cell lines, including AXL, TGFA, COLL7A1, and WNT5A. Three genes were overexpressed in the low metastatic cell line, including IL-16, MKK6, and BRAG [15]. In another mouse model of osteosarcoma using cell lines with different metastatic potential, 53 genes with differential expression were identified. These genes could be categorized into six general groups, including proliferation and apoptosis; motility and cytoskeleton; invasion; immune surveillance; adherence; and angiogenesis [16]. A separate microarray analysis of five metastatic human specimens demonstrated 13 genes that compared significantly to primary osteosarcomas [14].

Microarray analysis can also provide a method to analyze the effects of the single gene within an osteosarcoma cell line. A human osteosarcoma cell line was transfected with alkaline phosphatase gene. High and low expressing clones were selected. High expression of the alkaline phosphatase gene was associated with low metastatic potential. The addition of this one gene resulted in 79 differentially expressed genes. Alkaline phosphatase and 57 other genes were upregulated and 21 genes were downregulated. The differentially expressed genes could be grouped into categories, including cell growth and maintenance; cell cycle; signal transduction; DNA metabolism; RNA metabolism; cytoskeleton; and cell motility [17].

Microarray analysis has also been used to compare human osteosarcoma cells with normal human osteoblast. One such analysis demonstrated 35 differentially expressed genes with eight overexpressed and 27 underexpressed [18]. The differences in expression between tumor cell lines and the osteoblast were consistent for all cell lines. In a comparison of osteosarcoma in a long bone of a young patient with an atypical bone in an older patient, microarray analysis identified 15 genes that were able to segregate the specimens [13]. Recurrent osteosarcoma specimens have also been analyzed by microarray, demonstrating similar gene profiles between the primary and recurrent cases [14].

Growth factors

Several growth factor families have been implicated in normal development and in cancer. One such family is the Wingless-type (WNT) family of proteins that modulate cellular proliferation and embryogenesis. WNT proteins bind to cell surface receptors called frizzled (FZD) and LDL receptor–related proteins (LRP), leading to accumulation of cytoplasmic β-catenin. β-Catenin can then translocate into the nucleus and interact with transcription factor lymphoid enhancer factor (LEF) and T-cell factor to increase expression of WNT-responsive genes. These genes include cell cycle regulators, matrix-degrading enzymes, cytoskeletal proteins, and transcription factors. The WNT pathway has been implicated in skeletal development and in several human cancers. Multiple WNT and receptor family members have been identified in human osteosarcoma cell lines [19]. The LRP5 receptor was also identified in 50% of osteosarcoma specimens and its expression correlated significantly with metastatic events [19].

Her-2/neu is an epidermal growth factor receptor also known as ErbB2. It is a tyrosine kinase oncogene. Overexpression of Her-2/neu is related to poor prognosis in breast, ovarian, and lung cancers. Its expression is associated with tumor growth, invasion, and metastasis. The presence of Her-2/neu in osteosarcoma is controversial. Her-2/neu was not found in the serum of patients who had osteosarcoma [20]. Several studies have identified Her-2/neu expression in 42% to 63% of osteosarcomas [21]. A few studies have demonstrated expression to be associated with poorer response to chemotherapy and poorer overall survival, whereas others have shown that expression correlated with better survival [10,22]. Other studies have shown no significant expression of Her-2/neu in osteosarcoma [22]. Some of the discrepancy may be related to small sample size and different detection methods. However, as an antagonist for the Her-2/neu receptor already in use for carcinomas, Her-2/neu may represent an attractive therapeutic strategy.

In addition to growth factors, cytoskeletal proteins have also been implicated in tumor progression. Ezrin, a protein that facilitates linkage between the cell membrane, is also involved in signal transduction through the AKT and mitogen-activated protein kinase (MAPK) pathways [23]. Ezrin was first linked to osteosarcoma metastasis in a mouse model [16]. This protein has also been identified in human specimens and in spontaneous dog osteosarcomas [14]. In humans and dogs, ezrin is associated with a shorter disease-free interval [23].

Chemokines

Chemokines are a family of small, secreted proteins that are involved with leukocyte trafficking by interacting with cellular receptors. There are 18 different receptors identified, and they belong to the seven-transmembrane, G-coupled proteins [24]. Chemokine receptors have been associated with multiple types of malignant cancers, including breast, bladder, melanoma, colon, and lung [24,25]. Their presence has been correlated with poor prognosis, invasiveness, and the development of metastasis [24,25]. The chemokine receptor CXCR4 was found to be present in 63% of high-grade osteosarcoma specimens [25]. Its expression was inversely correlated with metastasis-free and overall survival [25]. Other chemokine receptors were also identified, including CCR10 and CCR7, but their relationship to metastasis and survival was less impressive [25].

Apoptosis

Fas (CD95 or APO-1) is a transmembrane receptor for FasL that induces apoptosis. Binding of FasL leads to trimerization of the receptors, causing the formation of the death-inducing signaling complex (DISC). The DISC leads to the activation of caspases that carry out apoptosis. Escape from Fas-induced apoptosis can be through decreased expression of Fas, FasL, or caspases, or increasing expression of bcl-2 and Fas associated death domain-like IL-1β converting enzyme (FLICE), a caspase inhibitor. For an osteosarcoma to have unregulated growth and metastasize to the lungs, it must escape the Fas/FasL-induced apoptosis. Human osteosarcoma cells selected for their ability to metastasize in a mouse model demonstrate decreased expression of Fas. If the expression of Fas is restored, this cell line has a lower potential to metastasize [26]. In those tumors with Fas, expression often correlates with necrotic areas [26].

IL-12 and IFN-γ have been shown to increase Fas expression [26,27]. FasL is expressed in the lungs and may be upregulated by ifosfamide [11,26]. Inducing IL-12 in a mouse model using human osteosarcoma cells lead to the reduction of pulmonary metastatic lesions. In a previous Intergroup Osteosarcoma Study, the combination of ifosfamide and MTP-PE, which can induce IL-12, showed a trend toward increased survival when both agents were administered. The induction of FasL by the ifosfamide and Fas by the MTP-PE/IL-12 was postulated as the explanation [11].

Transcription factors

For a sarcoma to have unlimited growth potential, it must not undergo terminal differentiation. Several transcription factors have been identified that are specific to the osteoblast lineage leading to mature osteoblast. These include osterix, runx2, and Dlx-5. Osterix is a zinc-fingered transcription factor that belongs to the SP family [28]. It appears to be critical for the development of mature osteoblasts and calcification of osseous tissues. Osterix expression in murine and human sarcoma cell lines was found to be significant below that of osteoblast. Cell lines that are transfected with osterix demonstrate a significant reduction in metastatic ability and the ability to form osteolytic primary tumors [29]. A second transcription factor required for osteoblast differentiation is runx2, which is a member of the runt family. Runx2 interacts with the Rb gene to the control cell cycle and the transcription levels of osteoblastic genes [30]. In human osteosarcoma cell lines, expression of runx2 is decreased compared with fibroblastic lines. Even when runx2 is present, its ability to stimulate transcription of osteoblastic genes appears decreased in osteosarcoma cell lines [30].

Chemotherapy resistance

Because chemotherapy has significantly improved the survival for osteosarcoma, patients who have tumors that are resistant to chemotherapy would be expected to have a poorer outcome. Several mechanisms are responsible for resistance to chemotherapy. P-glycoprotein, a product of the MDR1 gene, is an ATP-dependent efflux pump that may confer resistance to doxorubicin and etoposide [11]. Several studies have found P-glycoprotein in 30% to 40% of primary osteosarcomas [10,31]. In 19 patients who had primary tumors and pulmonary metastasis, the expression of P-glycoprotein was identified in 32% of primary tumors and 68% of metastasis. However, this did not correlate with event-free or overall survival [10]. This finding is in agreement with the osteosarcoma cooperative group phase 3 study, which did not find a significant difference in event-free or overall survival for P-glycoprotein expression [11]. However, evaluation of a large cohort of 149 patients found P-glycoprotein to be an indicator for event-free and overall survival [31]. However, P-glycoprotein expression was not correlated with tumor necrosis [31]. At this time, the role of P-glycoprotein in osteosarcoma chemotherapy resistance is unclear, but its expression may be a marker of tumor aggressiveness [11].

Another mechanism for resistance is the ability to inactivate chemotherapy agents. Cytochrome P450 oxidases are a large family of enzymes that are capable of inactivating many anticancer drugs, including etoposide, ifosfamide, and doxorubicin [32]. Immunohistochemical studies of biopsy specimens showed that the isoenzyme CYP3A4/5 was variably expressed in osteosarcoma and that higher expression correlated with development of metastasis and a poor outcome [32].

Angiogenesis

The development of metastasis is a complex process that requires multiple steps, one of which is the development of a stable blood supply. Before the advent of active chemotherapy agents, osteosarcoma patients often underwent immediate resection. A very high percentage of patients rapidly develop metastatic disease after their resections. Recent data in a mouse model may provide one explanation for the rapid development of metastatic disease after the primary tumor is removed. Mice subcutaneously inoculated with an osteosarcoma cell line developed primary tumors. When these primary tumors were resected, the animals developed more metastasis than if they had a sham operation. Although the level of vascular endothelial growth factor (VEGF) and its inhibitor endostatin were lower after tumor resection, the angiogenesis inhibitor TNP-470 still blocked the formation of metastatic lesions [33]. In human patients who had osteosarcoma, those who developed a pulmonary metastasis after removal of the primary tumor had significantly higher levels of VEGF and endostatin than those who do not develop metastasis.

The postoperative change for the patients in the recurrence group showed a much more dramatic drop for endostatin than for VEGF [34]. Though VEGF was reduced, it may have significant angiogenic effects after the inhibitory effect of endostatin was removed.

Interstitial pressure

Solid tumors such as osteosarcoma maintain high levels of intratumoral interstitial pressure. Recent experiments on the effects of interstitial fluid pressure on osteosarcoma cells yielded interesting results. Cells grown under pressure exhibit more proliferation when measured by cell cycle analysis [35]. In addition, pressurized osteosarcoma cells showed increased chemosensitivity to doxorubicin and cisplatin. Clinically, tumors with higher interstitial fluid pressure exhibited a higher degree of histologic necrosis [35]. These results suggest that pressurized culture system may afford more physiologically relevant studies of osteosarcoma biology in the future.

Summary

With the advent of chemotherapy, the treatment for osteosarcoma has made significant progress. However, this progress has slowed in recent years, leaving approximately 30% to 40% of patients who will do poorly. Research has been focused on identifying these patients early and elucidating new pathways that serve as targets for therapy. Microarray analysis is providing new means for patient risk stratification and identifying new molecules that may serve as therapeutic targets. Newly identified genes that are important for growth and development, such as the WNT/LRP5 pathway, are being investigated for their role in osteosarcoma. Chemokines may play a role in stimulating the invasiveness and homing of metastatic disease. Cytoskeletal proteins such as ezrin reveal their critical role in promoting tumor metastasis. Genes involved oncogenesis and apoptosis in other malignant tumors are being evaluated, such as Her-2/neu and Fas. Studies of osteosarcoma cells under a pressurized environment may yield important clues about tumor proliferation and responses to chemotherapy. With lessons learned from other cancers and improved molecular techniques, osteosarcoma will eventually reveal much of its secrets, yielding new ways to categorize patients and treat this disease more effectively.

References

[1] Bielack SS, Kempf-Bielack B, Delling G, et al. Prognostic factors in high-grade osteosarcoma of the extremities or trunk: an analysis of 1,702 patients treated on neoadjuvant cooperative osteosarcoma study group protocols. J Clin Oncol 2002;20:776–90.

[2] Picci P, Ferrari S, Bacci G, et al. Treatment recommendations for osteosarcoma and adult soft tissue sarcomas. Drugs 1994;47:82–92.

[3] Hauben EI, Weeden S, Pringle J, et al. Does the histological subtype of high-grade central osteosarcoma influence the response to treatment with chemotherapy and does it affect overall survival? A study on 570 patients of two consecutive trials of the European Osteosarcoma Intergroup. Eur J Cancer 2002;38: 1218–25.

[4] Kempf-Bielack B, Bielack SS, Jurgens H, et al. Osteosarcoma relapse after combined modality therapy: an analysis of unselected patients in the Cooperative Osteosarcoma Study Group (COSS). J Clin Oncol 2005;23:559–68.

[5] Meyers PA. High-dose therapy with autologous stem cell rescue for pediatric sarcomas. Curr Opin Oncol 2004;16:120–5.

[6] Ross JA, Davies SM. Childhood cancer etiology: recent reports. Med Pediatr Oncol 2001;37:55–8.

[7] Buckley JD, Pendergrass TW, Buckley CM, et al. Epidemiology of osteosarcoma and Ewing's sarcoma in childhood: a study of 305 cases by the Children's Cancer Group. Cancer 1998;83:1440–8.

[8] Fuchs B, Pritchard DJ. Etiology of osteosarcoma. Clin Orthop Relat Res 2002;397:40–52.

[9] Wunder JS, Gokgoz N, Parkes R, et al. TP53 mutations and outcome in osteosarcoma: a prospective, multicenter study. J Clin Oncol 2005;23:1483–90.

[10] Ferrari S, Bertoni F, Zanella L, et al. Evaluation of P-glycoprotein, HER-2/ErbB-2, p53, and Bcl-2 in primary tumor and metachronous lung metastases in patients with high-grade osteosarcoma. Cancer 2004; 100:1936–42.

[11] Gorlick R, Anderson P, Andrulis I, et al. Biology of childhood osteogenic sarcoma and potential targets for therapeutic development: meeting summary. Clin Cancer Res 2003;9:5442–53.

[12] Mintz MB, Sowers R, Brown KM, et al. An expression signature classifies chemotherapy-resistant pediatric osteosarcoma. Cancer Res 2005;65:1748–54.

[13] Ochi K, Daigo Y, Katagiri T, et al. Prediction of response to neoadjuvant chemotherapy for osteosarcoma by gene-expression profiles. Int J Oncol 2004;24:647–55.

[14] Leonard P, Sharp T, Henderson S, et al. Gene expression array profile of human osteosarcoma. Br J Cancer 2003;89:2284–8.

[15] Nakano T, Tani M, Ishibashi Y, et al. Biological properties and gene expression associated with metastatic potential of human osteosarcoma. Clin Exp Metastasis 2003;20:665–74.

[16] Khanna C, Khan J, Nguyen P, et al. Metastasis-associated differences in gene expression in a murine model of osteosarcoma. Cancer Res 2001;61:3750–9.

[17] Zucchini C, Bianchini M, Valvassori L, et al. Identification of candidate genes involved in the reversal of malignant phenotype of osteosarcoma cells transfected with the liver/bone/kidney alkaline phosphatase gene. Bone 2004;34:672–9.

[18] Wolf M, El-Rifai W, Tarkkanen M, et al. Novel findings in gene expression detected in human osteosarcoma by cDNA microarray. Cancer Genet Cytogenet 2000;123:128–32.

[19] Hoang BH, Kubo T, Healey JH, et al. Expression of LDL receptor-related protein 5 (LRP5) as a novel marker for disease progression in high-grade osteosarcoma. Int J Cancer 2004;109:106–11.

[20] Holzer G, Pfandlsteiner T, Koschat M, et al. Soluble p185(HER-2) in patients with malignant bone tumours. Pediatr Blood Cancer 2005;44:163–8.

[21] Zhou H, Randall RL, Brothman AR, et al. Her-2/neu expression in osteosarcoma increases risk of lung metastasis and can be associated with gene amplification. J Pediatr Hematol Oncol 2003;25:27–32.

[22] Anninga JK, van de Vijver MJ, Cleton-Jansen AM, et al. Overexpression of the HER-2 oncogene does not play a role in high-grade osteosarcomas. Eur J Cancer 2004;40:963–70.

[23] Khanna C, Wan X, Bose S, et al. The membrane-cytoskeleton linker ezrin is necessary for osteosarcoma metastasis. Nat Med 2004;10:182–6.

[24] Retz MM, Sidhu SS, Blaveri E, et al. CXCR4 expression reflects tumor progression and regulates motility of bladder cancer cells. Int J Cancer 2005; 114:182–9.

[25] Laverdiere C, Hoang BH, Yang R, et al. Messenger RNA expression levels of CXCR4 correlate with metastatic behavior and outcome in patients with osteosarcoma. Clin Cancer Res 2005;11:2561–7.

[26] Lafleur EA, Koshkina NV, Stewart J, et al. Increased Fas expression reduces the metastatic potential of human osteosarcoma cells. Clin Cancer Res 2004; 10:8114–9.

[27] Inaba H, Glibetic M, Buck S, et al. Interferon-gamma sensitizes osteosarcoma cells to Fas-induced apoptosis by up-regulating Fas receptors and caspase-8. Pediatr Blood Cancer 2004;43:729–36.

[28] Nakashima K, Zhou X, Kunkel G, et al. The novel zinc finger-containing transcription factor osterix is required for osteoblast differentiation and bone formation. Cell 2002;108:17–29.

[29] Cao Y, Zhou Z, de Crombrugghe B, et al. Osterix, a transcription factor for osteoblast differentiation, mediates antitumor activity in murine osteosarcoma. Cancer Res 2005;65:1124–8.

[30] Thomas DM, Johnson SA, Sims NA, et al. Terminal osteoblast differentiation, mediated by runx2 and p27KIP1, is disrupted in osteosarcoma. J Cell Biol 2004;167:925–34.

[31] Serra M, Scotlandi K, Reverter-Branchat G, et al. Value of P-glycoprotein and clinicopathologic factors

as the basis for new treatment strategies in high-grade osteosarcoma of the extremities. J Clin Oncol 2003; 21:536–42.

[32] Dhaini HR, Thomas DG, Giordano TJ, et al. Cytochrome P450 CYP3A4/5 expression as a biomarker of outcome in osteosarcoma. J Clin Oncol 2003;21: 2481–95.

[33] Tsunemi T, Nagoya S, Kaya M, et al. Postoperative progression of pulmonary metastasis in osteosarcoma. Clin Orthop Relat Res 2003;407:159–66.

[34] Kaya M, Wada T, Nagoya S, et al. Concomitant tumour resistance in patients with osteosarcoma. A clue to a new therapeutic strategy. J Bone Joint Surg Br 2004; 86:143–7.

[35] Nathan SS, DiResta GR, Casas-Ganem JE, et al. Elevated physiologic tumor pressure promotes proliferation and chemosensitivity in human osteosarcoma. Clin Cancer Res 2005;11:2389–97.

ELSEVIER
SAUNDERS

Orthop Clin N Am 37 (2006) 9 – 14

ORTHOPEDIC
CLINICS
OF NORTH AMERICA

Recent Advances in the Basic Science of Chondrosarcoma

Richard M. Terek, MD

Department of Orthopedic Surgery, Brown University, UOI, MOC, Suite 200, 2 Dudley Street, Providence, RI 02905, USA

Chondrosarcoma are primary bone tumors that bear some relationship to the cartilage phenotype. They can arise de novo (primary) or from a preexisting benign cartilage tumors, such as an enchondroma or osteochondroma (secondary). Conventional chondrosarcoma are graded as I, II, and III. In addition, there are specialized types of chondrosarcoma that include clear cell, mesenchymal, dedifferentiated, and myxoid. The molecular underpinnings of some of these tumors may overlap. There may be an orderly progression of acquired molecular abnormalities advancing from grade I to III. More likely, however, is that each should be studied individually because on balance, chondrosarcoma appear to be a heterogeneous group of neoplasms.

Strategies to identify the molecular underpinnings of a tumor include cytogenetics, comparative genomics, and the candidate gene approach. The first two are broad screening approaches that frequently identify a large number of abnormalities, some of which may play a role in the pathophysiology of the tumor. The candidate gene approach is a detailed analysis of a single gene that may start with an analysis of expression of a gene in a tumor and its corresponding normal tissue. Proof that a gene actually is part of the pathophysiology requires techniques of functional genomics that include introducing an expression vector for a normal or mutated gene into a cell or blocking the expression of a gene and observing the effect on one of the phenotypes associated with malignancy, such as proliferation or invasion. Stronger proof requires use of transgenic or knockout mice. Candidate genes are put forth based on knowledge about normal cell biology,

other tumors, genes identified using aforementioned screening techniques, and embryology—embryology because one principle seems to be that some genes transiently expressed during normal growth and development are reactivated in tumors, which can impart a selective advantage to the tumor cell. The concept that the pathophysiology of cancer may involve the reactivation of pathways that are normally active only during normal growth and development raises the question of whether the pathophysiolgy of chondrosarcoma is related to the cartilaginous phenotype or the growth plate [1].

Though it is straightforward to analyze the effect of reexpression of a single gene or the effect of a single gene mutation, it is more difficult to study the effects of multiple genetic abnormalities and more subtle abnormalities that go beyond the digital paradigm of a gene being "on" or "off." Pathology can result from abnormal levels of gene expression, abnormal timing of expression, and abnormalities in shuttling of proteins between the cytoplasm and nucleus. And this says nothing of the extent to which any of these abnormalities are influenced by the context in which they occur (eg, the immune status of the host).

The basic characteristics of a malignant tumor are unrestrained growth and the ability to metastasize. The development of a tumor with the ability to metastasize is a multistep process that entails the accumulation of at least several genetic changes. As cells become genetically unstable, there is selective pressure for those cells that have the greatest growth advantage, not unlike selecting out resistant bacteria in culture. It has been proposed that these genetic changes fall into one of six categories, each of which describes a facet of tumor physiology [2]: (1) self-sufficiency in growth signals; (2) insensitivity to

---

E-mail address: Richard_Terek@Brown.edu

growth inhibitory signals; (3) evasion of programmed cell death (apoptosis); (4) limitless replicative potential; (5) sustained angiogenesis; and (6) tissue invasion and metastasis.

The following review starts with genetic screening techniques that have been used to study chondrosarcoma. Specific abnormalities will be organized according to the six categories in the preceding paragraph as well as those having to do with treatment response.

Cytogenetics

Cytogenetic analysis of chondrosarcoma have shown an extreme heterogeneity of findings [3,4]. Cytogenetic abnormalities include missing and duplicated chromosomes, deletions and duplications of portions of chromosomes, and translocations. One tumor may have all of these abnormalities. Though there is some clustering of chromosomal regions affected by abnormalities, it has been difficult to get clues from the cytogenetics about which genes or pathways are aberrantly expressed in these tumors.

Self-sufficiency in growth signals

One example of a cytogenetic abnormality that has proven useful and is an exception to the previous statement is the translocation between chromosomes 9 and 22 found in at least 75% of extraskeletal myxoid chondrosarcoma (EMC) [3,4]. The translocation results in a fusion of the *EWS* and *TEC* genes. This translocation results in a fusion protein with oncogenic properties. *EWS* is an RNA binding protein, and *TEC* is a putative orphan nuclear receptor (part of the thyroid and steroid receptor family) that also has a DNA binding domain. The exact splice point between the two genes can occur at two different locations, but the end result is the activation of genes by *TEC* having to do with cell proliferation. Translocations found in the remaining 25% of EMC involve alternatives to *EWS*: *TAF2N/TEC* and *TCF12/TEC*. The biologic activity of these splicing variants may differ, and therefore their analysis may allow for more precise prognostication and provide for unique therapeutic targets.

Insensitivity to growth inhibitory signals

Hereditary multiple exostoses (HME) is an autosomal dominant disorder characterized by multiple osteochondromas. Linkage analysis has resulted in the cloning of three genes related to this disease:

EXT1, EXT2, and EXT3. Most patients have inactivating mutations in EXT1 or EXT2. The mutations include deletions, splicing errors, missense, and frameshift. The proteins coded for by these genes are glycosyltransferases involved in the biosynthesis of heparan sulfate proteoglycans [5].

More severe disease and a higher risk of malignant transformation are associated with mutations in EXT1 [6]. Loss of function leading to abnormal growth technically places these genes in the category of a tumor suppressor gene. Heparan sulfate proteoglycans bind and create gradients of Indian hedgehog (IHH), paraththyroid related protein (PThRP), and fibroblast growth factor (FGF), all of which are involved with cartilage growth and maturation. The implication is that loss of a binding protein for growth regulating proteins because of an upstream mutation in an enzyme (EXT) results in abnormal growth.

The IHH/PThRP axis has been implicated in multiple enchondromatosis and potentially the development of chondrosarcoma. In the growth plate, IHH maintains chondrocytes in the proliferative phase, and PThRP downregulates IHH. Mutations in the receptor for PThRP have been found in some patients with multiple enchondromas and presumably inactivate this pathway resulting in persistence of the proliferating phase and the formation of enchondromas. A transgenic mouse model with PThRP receptor mutation results in just such a phenotype [7], and a mouse with a mutation in *GLI1*, a protein which downregulates IHH, has a predispositon to synovial chondromatosis [8], leading the investigators to propose IHH blocking compounds as therapy for cartilaginous neoplasms [8,9].

Other reports implicate more traditional suppressor genes, such as p16 [10,11] and p53 [12], in the progression of chondrosarcoma to the higher grades, although results for the latter are inconsistent [11,13].

Evasion of programmed cell death (apoptosis)

PTHrP is known to regulate chondrocyte maturation in the growth plate. Associated with maturation is apoptosis, which is regulated by the ratio of *Bcl-2/Bax* gene expression. *Bax* counteracts the antiapoptotic effect of *Bcl-2*. Both PTHrP and *Bcl-2* were found in higher levels in malignant compared with benign cartilage tumors, and there was a correlation with grade [14,15]. Treatment of a human chondrosarcoma cell line with monoclonal antibodies directed against PTHrP resulted in an increase in apoptosis, a decrease in *Bcl-2*, an increase in *Bax*, and, counterintuitively, maturation of the chondrosarcoma cells as evidenced by an increase in expression of collagen type X, which is associated with hypertrophic chondrocytes [16]. These results are also somewhat contradictory in that loss of the inhibitory effect of PTHrP on IHH expression is supposed to result in cartilage tumors, whereas in this study blocking PTHrP signaling was beneficial.

Limitless replicative potential

Most cells have a limited number of doublings, after which there is replicative senescence, which results from progressive shortening of the tips of chromosomes after each mitotic event. Tumor cells reactivate telomerase, which restores the nucleotides lost at the tips of chromosomes with mitosis. The studies of telomerase activity in chondrosarcoma are not consistent. One study found no increase in telomerase activity in chondrosarcoma compared with benign cartilage lesions, and found telomerase inhibitory activity in tumor lysates [17]. Other investigators have found telomerase activity in chondrosarcoma and also that telomerase activity increases with serial passaging of chondrosarcoma cells in culture from tumors that initially did not have telomerase activity [18]. A follow-up study found that telomerase expression was associated with tumor grade and recurrence [19].

Sustained angiogenesis

Angiogenesis, the formation of new blood vessels, is a tightly regulated process that occurs during wound and fracture healing, normal growth and development, pregnancy, and growth of neoplasms [20,21]. The two most important traits of cancer are unrestrained growth and development of metastases [2]. Diffusion of adequate amounts of oxygen for aerobic cellular metabolism is limited to 200 μm, so that once a tumor grows beyond several millimeters, angiogenesis must occur to support further growth. The first step in metastasis is for the tumor cell to gain access to the circulation. Neovessels are considered leaky and allow for tumor cell egress into the circulation. Once in the circulation, some tumor cells can adhere and begin growth in another location. The ability to induce sustained angiogenesis is a necessary condition for both of these traits [2]. Angiogenesis therefore plays a central role in both of the two most important traits of neoplasia. Virtually all of the research on tumor vascularity and the known factors that stimulate angiogenesis have shown a correlation between vascularity,

expression of proangiogenic factors, biologic aggressiveness, high pathologic grade, and poor survival [22]. Thus if one could interrupt tumor angiogenesis one might be able to decrease tumor growth and metastasis [23,24]. Vascularity has only been recently evaluated in chondrosarcoma. One could argue that chondrosarcoma are less likely to be vascular because of their relationship to cartilage, which is avascular. Alternatively, one could argue that they are just as likely to be vascular because chondrosarcoma can be large bulky tumors that must become hypoxic. Microvascular density was determined using immunohistochemistry on a spectrum of conventional chondrosarcoma and benign cartilage lesions. Grade II and III chondrosarcomas had the same microvascular density, which was 4.5 times more than benign or grade I tumors [25]. Microvascularity correlates with clinical behavior because it is primarily grade II and III chondrosarcomas that metastasize. Thus, chondrosarcoma development is linked to angiogenesis.

The prime stimulus for angiogenesis is hypoxia. Hypoxia results in increased protein levels of the transcription factor hypoxia-inducible factor-1 (HIF-1) [26]. HIF-1 is a nuclear protein that activates gene transcription in response to reduced oxygen tension. HIF-1 is a heterodimer composed of HIF-1α and HIF-1β subunits. HIF-1β is constitutively expressed, whereas HIF-1α is induced by hypoxia. The regulation of HIF-1α occurs at the transcriptional, translational, nuclear translocation, and transactivation steps. During normoxia, HIF-1α is degraded. During hypoxia, degradation ceases and HIF-1α accumulates. The HIF-1 heterodimer, acting in conjunction with the coactivator proteins CBP, p300, SRC-1, and TIF2, increases expression of genes related to glycolysis and angiogenesis. The most important angiogenic cytokine activated by HIF-1 is VEGF [12], which alleviates the hypoxic condition by stimulating vascular ingrowth. Analysis of HIF-1α expression in chondrosarcoma tissue with immunohistochemistry has shown that the more vascularized tumors (grade II and III) have more staining for this transcription factor [27]. Analogous to HIF-1α, VEGF was expressed at a higher level in the angiogenic group compared with the nonangiogenic group [27].

Under normoxic conditions, HIF-1α is degraded. Under hypoxic conditions, degradation is inhibited, and HIF-1α protein accumulates. To determine if HIF expression in chondrosarcoma was at least in part a physiologic response to hypoxia, Western blotting was performed to detect expression of this transcription factor in chondrosarcoma cell lines and normal chondrocytes cultured under normoxic and hypoxic conditions. Chondrosarcoma cell lines and normal chondrocytes all express HIF-1α under hypoxic conditions, indicating that the cartilage phenotype does not result in loss of hypoxia-inducible pathways. Therefore, hypoxia induced HIF-1α expression is consistent with the hypothesis that hypoxia is a driving force behind angiogenic activity in chondrosarcoma. Presumably, normal cartilage and low-grade chondrosarcoma have such a low metabolic and proliferative rate that they do not become as hypoxic as a growing tumor, and therefore angiogenic pathways are not activated in vivo. Another explanation for this lack of angiogenesis in normal cartilage and low-grade chondosarcoma is the presence of angiogenic inhibitors.

Blocking expression of hypoxia-induced HIF-1α using the strategy of short inhibitory RNA sequences complementary to HIF-1α resulted in a marked inhibition of hypoxia-induced upregulation of VEGF mRNA, suggesting that HIF-1a may be an appropriate antiangiogenic target [28].

In an analysis of HIF-1α, VEGF, and bFGF expression in Swarm rat chondrosarcoma, it was found that HIF-1α and VEGF levels were increased in avascular tumors and then decreased in the angiogenic tumor nodules. The explanation given is that initially the tumor nodules are avascular and therefore hypoxic, resulting in expression of HIF-1α and VEGF. After the nodules are vascularized, they are no longer hypoxic and expression of these factors goes down, suggesting that HIF-1α and VEGF mediate the angiogenic switch [29]. In contrast, bFGF levels increased in the angiogenic nodules, leading to the interpretation that bFGF is not involved with angiogenesis, but more likely related to tumor growth.

Because cartilage is avascular, it has been long suspected and subsequently proven to contain inhibitors of angiogenesis [30]. Some proteins that have been identified are chondromodulin I (ChM-I) [31], troponin I (TnI) [32], plasminogen-related protein B [33], TIMP-1,2,3, and thrombospondin-1. ChM-I is present in the avascular portion of the growth plate, and its expression is absent from the late hypertrophic and calcified portions of the growth plate. The latter areas are where cartilage becomes vascularized as part of the endochondral ossification process. ChMI has inhibitory effects on vascular endothelial cells and is a glycosylated, secreted protein found primarily in the interterritorial space of the matrix [34]. Cartilage is known to contain proangiogenic factors such as VEGF, bFGF, and TGF-beta, suggesting that ChM-I and other antiangiogenic proteins are able to counteract these molecules [34]. The human

sequence of ChMI was determined from expression of the gene in grade I chondrosarcoma, which are less vascular than grade II and III chondrosarcomas [25]. Recombinant human ChM-I has been made and shown to inhibit tube formation by cultured vascular endothelial cells and inhibit angiogenesis in the chick chorioallantoic membrane [35]. Thus, ChM-I is an antiangiogenic molecule.

Besides ChMI, there are other antiangiogenic molecules found in cartilage, although their expression is not limited to cartilage as is ChMI. Troponin I (TnI) was identified as an endogenous angiogenesis inhibitor in cartilage by screening protein extracts from cartilage for their ability to inhibit proliferation of endothelial cells stimulated by bFGF [32].

Plasminogen related protein B has antiangiogenic properties. When tested in combination with ecteinascidin-743, a marine-derived chemotherapeutic agent against chondrosarcoma cell lines in vitro and in vivo, the results were synergistic with respect to tumor necrosis and inhibition of neovascularity [36]. The idea of combining a traditional cytotoxic chemotherapeutic agent with a cytostatic antiangiogenic agent has proven fruitful for treating other types of tumors as well.

Tissue invasion and metastasis

The ability of a tumor cell to invade and transgress tissue boundaries is in part related to angiogenesis in that both processes require the expression of matrix metalloproteinases. The matrix metalloproteinases are a family of at least 20 enzymes, each of which can degrade extracellular matrix proteins. The activity of the metalloproteinases is determined by the ratio of these enzymes to their respective tissue inhibitors of metalloproteinases (TIMPs). The ratio of MMP-1/TIMP-1 was correlated with recurrent disease and poor survival [37]. Subsequent studies have shown that MMP-1 gene expression could be knocked down in human chondrosarcoma cells with siRNA, resulting in decreased levels and activity of MMP-1 and decreased invasiveness in vitro [38–40]. Both TIMP2 and 3 have been shown to have antiangiogenic properties through an MMP-independent mechanism [41], and TIMP-3 expression was able to inhibit tumor growth and angiogenesis in neuroblastoma [42].

Response to treatment

Chondrosarcoma are considered resistant to chemotherapy. Previous studies suggested that chemoresistance to drugs such as doxorubicin might be related to expression of the multidrug resistant-1 gene (MDR-1) [43–45]. MDR-1 codes for p-glycoprotein, a transmembrane protein capable of transporting some chemotherapeutic agents out of the cell. A more recent study has shown that resistance to ecteinascidin-743 is mediated by a non-MDR mechanism, related to rearrangement of the actin cytoskeleton [46]. A gene chip analysis comparing the resistant to parent cell line identified 70 genes associated with the resistant phenotype, indicating the complexity of molecular abnormalities that underlie any phenotypic trait.

Summary

The pathophysiology of chondrosarcoma is complex. Advances in our understanding of this tumor at the molecular levels are improving. Efforts at understanding the relationship of chondrosarcoma to the growth plate and benign cartilage lesions have been fruitful. The rarity of higher-grade tumors reinforces the need for multi-institutional cooperative studies with long-term follow-up and multivariate analysis of traditional clinical and histopathologic parameters in conjunction with molecular abnormalities identified through gene chip analysis. Advances in molecular targeting of therapeutics are necessary to improve the fate of patients with chondrosarcoma.

References

[1] Bovee JV, Cleton-Jansen AM, Taminiau AH, et al. Emerging pathways in the development of chondrosarcoma of bone and implications for targeted treatment. Lancet Oncol 2005;6(8):599–607.

[2] Hanahan D, Weinberg RA. The hallmarks of cancer. Cell 2000;100(1):57–70.

[3] Sandberg AA. Genetics of chondrosarcoma and related tumors. Curr Opin Oncol 2004;16(4):342–54.

[4] Sandberg AA, Bridge JA. Updates on the cytogenetics and molecular genetics of bone and soft tissue tumors: chondrosarcoma and other cartilaginous neoplasms. Cancer Genet Cytogenet 2003;143(1):1–31.

[5] Francannet C, Cohen-Tanugi A, Le Merrer M, et al. Genotype-phenotype correlation in hereditary multiple exostoses. J Med Genet 2001;38(7):430–4.

[6] Porter DE, Lonie L, Fraser M, et al. Severity of disease and risk of malignant change in hereditary multiple exostoses. A genotype-phenotype study. J Bone Joint Surg [Br] 2004;86(7):1041–6.

[7] Hopyan S, Gokgoz N, Poon R, et al. A mutant PTH/PTHrP type I receptor in enchondromatosis. Nat Genet 2002;30(3):306–10.

[8] Hopyan S, Nadesan P, Yu C, et al. Dysregulation of hedgehog signalling predisposes to synovial chondromatosis. J Pathol 2005;206(2):143–50.

[9] Tiet TD, Alman BA. Developmental pathways in musculoskeletal neoplasia: involvement of the Indian Hedgehog-parathyroid hormone-related protein pathway. Pediatr Res 2003;53(4):539–43.

[10] van Beerendonk HM, Rozeman LB, Taminiau AH, et al. Molecular analysis of the INK4A/INK4A-ARF gene locus in conventional (central) chondrosarcomas and enchondromas: indication of an important gene for tumour progression. J Pathol 2004;202(3):359–66.

[11] Asp J, Sangiorgi L, Inerot SE, et al. Changes of the p16 gene but not the p53 gene in human chondrosarcoma tissues. Int J Cancer 2000;85(6):782–6.

[12] Ferrara N, Davis-Smyth T. The biology of vascular endothelial growth factor. Endocr Rev 1997;18(1):4–25.

[13] Terek RM, Healey JH, Garin-Chesa P, et al. p53 mutations in chondrosarcoma. Diagn Mol Pathol 1998;7(1):51–6.

[14] Amling M, Posl M, Hentz MW, et al. PTHrP and Bcl-2: essential regulatory molecules in chondrocyte differentiation and chondrogenic tumors. Verh Dtsch Ges Pathol 1998;82:160–9.

[15] Bovee JV, van Den Broek LJ, Cleton-Jansen AM, et al. Up-regulation of PTHrP and Bcl-2 expression characterizes the progression of osteochondroma towards peripheral chondrosarcoma and is a late event in central chondrosarcoma. Lab Invest 2000;80(12):1925–34.

[16] Miyaji T, Nakase T, Onuma E, et al. Monoclonal antibody to parathyroid hormone-related protein induces differentiation and apoptosis of chondrosarcoma cells. Cancer Lett 2003;199(2):147–55.

[17] Bovee JV, van Den Broek LJ, Cleton-Jansen AM, et al. Chondrosarcoma is not characterized by detectable telomerase activity. J Pathol 2001;193(3):354–60.

[18] Rofstad EK. Microenvironment-induced cancer metastasis. Int J Radiat Biol 2000;76(5):589–605.

[19] Martin JA, DeYoung BR, Gitelis S, et al. Telomerase reverse transcriptase subunit expression is associated with chondrosarcoma malignancy. Clin Orthop Relat Res 2004;426:117–24.

[20] Kerbel RS. Tumor angiogenesis: past, present and the near future. Carcinogenesis 2000;21(3):505–15.

[21] Hanahan D, Folkman J. Patterns and emerging mechanisms of the angiogenic switch during tumorigenesis. Cell 1996;86(3):353–64.

[22] Weidner N, Semple JP, Welch WR, et al. Tumor angiogenesis and metastasis—correlation in invasive breast carcinoma. N Engl J Med 1991;324(1):1–8.

[23] Folkman J. Tumor angiogenesis: therapeutic implications. N Engl J Med 1971;285(21):1182–6.

[24] Folkman J. Fighting cancer by attacking its blood supply. Sci Am 1996;275(3):150–4.

[25] McGough RL, Aswad BI, Terek RM. Pathologic neovascularization in cartilage tumors. Clin Orthop 2002;397:76–82.

[26] Maxwell PH, Pugh CW, Ratcliffe PJ. Activation of the HIF pathway in cancer. Curr Opin Genet Dev 2001; 11(3):293 – 9.

[27] McGough RL, Lin C, Meitner P, et al. Angiogenic cytokines in cartilage tumors. Clin Orthop Relat Res 2002;397:62 – 9.

[28] Lin C, McGough R, Aswad B, et al. Hypoxia induces HIF-1alpha and VEGF expression in chondrosarcoma cells and chondrocytes. J Orthop Res 2004;22(6): 1175 – 81.

[29] Fang J, Yan L, Shing Y, et al. HIF-1alpha-mediated up-regulation of vascular endothelial growth factor, independent of basic fibroblast growth factor, is important in the switch to the angiogenic phenotype during early tumor genesis. Cancer Res 2001;61(15): 5731 – 5.

[30] Brem H, Folkman J. Inhibition of tumor angiogenesis mediated by cartilage. J Exp Med 1975;141(2): 427 – 39.

[31] Hiraki Y, Mitsui K, Endo N, et al. Molecular cloning of human chondromodulin-I, a cartilage-derived growth modulating factor, and its expression in Chinese hamster ovary cells. Eur J Biochem 1999;260(3): 869 – 78.

[32] Moses MA, Wiederschain D, Wu I, et al. Troponin I is present in human cartilage and inhibits angiogenesis. Proc Natl Acad Sci USA 1999;96(6):2645 – 50.

[33] Weissbach L, Treadwell BV. A plasminogen-related gene is expressed in cancer cells. Biochem Biophys Res Commun 1992;186(2):1108 – 14.

[34] Hiraki Y, Shukunami C. Chondromodulin-I as a novel cartilage-specific growth-modulating factor. Pediatr Nephrol 2000;14(7):602 – 5.

[35] Hiraki Y, Mitsui K, Endo N, et al. Molecular cloning of human chondromodulin-I, a cartilage-derived growth modulating factor, and its expression in Chinese hamster ovary cells. Eur J Biochem 1999;260(3): 869 – 78.

[36] Morioka H, Weissbach L, Vogel T, et al. Antiangiogenesis treatment combined with chemotherapy produces chondrosarcoma necrosis. Clin Cancer Res 2003;9(3):1211 – 7.

[37] Berend KR, Toth AP, Harrelson JM, et al. Association between ratio of matrix metalloproteinase-1 to tissue inhibitor of metalloproteinase-1 and local recurrence, metastasis, and survival in human chondrosarcoma. J Bone Joint Surg [Am] 1998;80(1):11 – 7.

[38] Yuan J, Dutton CM, Scully SP. RNAi mediated MMP-1 silencing inhibits human chondrosarcoma invasion. J Orthop Res 2005, in press.

[39] Jiang X, Dutton CM, Qi W, et al. Inhibition of MMP-1 expression by antisense RNA decreases invasiveness of human chondrosarcoma. J Orthop Res 2003;21(6): 1063 – 70.

[40] Jiang X, Dutton CM, Qi WN, et al. siRNA mediated inhibition of MMP-1 reduces invasive potential of a human chondrosarcoma cell line. J Cell Physiol 2005; 202(3):723 – 30.

[41] Seo DW, Li H, Guedez L, et al. TIMP-2 mediated inhibition of angiogenesis: an MMP-independent mechanism. Cell 2003;114(2):171 – 80.

[42] Spurbeck WW, Ng CY, Vanin EF, et al. Retroviral vector-producer cell-mediated in vivo gene transfer of TIMP-3 restricts angiogenesis and neuroblastoma growth in mice. Cancer Gene Ther 2003;10(3):161 – 7.

[43] Terek RM, Schwartz GK, Devaney K, et al. Chemotherapy and P-glycoprotein expression in chondrosarcoma. J Orthop Res 1998;16(5):585 – 90.

[44] Wyman JJ, Hornstein AM, Meitner PA, et al. Multidrug resistance-1 and p-glycoprotein in human chondrosarcoma cell lines: expression correlates with decreased intracellular doxorubicin and in vitro chemoresistance. J Orthop Res 1999;17(6):935 – 40.

[45] Rosier RN, O'Keefe RJ, Teot LA, et al. P-glycoprotein expression in cartilaginous tumors. J Surg Oncol 1997; 65(2):95 – 105.

[46] Shao L, Kasanov J, Hornicek FJ, et al. Ecteinascidin-743 drug resistance in sarcoma cells: transcriptional and cellular alterations. Biochem Pharmacol 2003; 66(12):2381 – 95.

ELSEVIER
SAUNDERS

Orthop Clin N Am 37 (2006) 15 – 22

ORTHOPEDIC
CLINICS
OF NORTH AMERICA

Advances in Chemotherapy for Patients with Extremity Soft Tissue Sarcoma

Fritz C. Eilber, MD*, William D. Tap, MD, Scott D. Nelson, MD,
Jeffery J. Eckardt, MD, Frederick R. Eilber, MD

University of California, Los Angeles, UCLA Medical Center, 10833 Le Conte Avenue, Los Angeles, CA 90095-1782, USA

Throughout the past several decades, chemotherapy (neoadjuvant or adjuvant) has been used in an attempt to improve the outcome of patients who have localized soft tissue sarcomas. These efforts have predominately been focused on the treatment of patients who have high-risk primary extremity soft tissue sarcomas, as they have a considerable risk for harboring subclinical micrometastasis at presentation [1,2]. Through the analysis of large sarcoma databases, high-risk extremity soft tissue sarcomas have become specifically defined as large (> 5 cm), deep, high-grade tumors (American Joint Committee on Cancer [AJCC] stage III) [3]. Patients who have such tumors have a 5-year disease-specific mortality of up to or greater than 50% [3–8]. The combination of proper oncologic surgery and radiation therapy has been successful in achieving excellent local control and functional results in these patients. Local recurrence rates for patients who have primary disease are about 10%, with less than 5% requiring amputation [7–9]. Despite improvements in local control and advances in limb salvage, the development of distant metastasis remains a significant problem, limiting the survival of patients who have high-risk extremity soft tissue sarcomas.

From the mid-1970s to the early 1990s, doxorubicin-based chemotherapy (DOX) was the most widely employed chemotherapeutic treatment for adult soft tissue sarcomas. Its impact on patients who have localized soft tissue sarcomas is summa-

rized by a meta-analysis of 14 randomized trials (1568 patients) comparing DOX to no chemotherapy [10]. Although there was a statistically significant (10%) improvement in recurrence-free survival for patients treated with DOX, there was not a significant improvement in overall survival (4%) (Fig. 1). A subset analysis of 886 patients who had extremity soft tissue sarcomas found a small (7%) but significant improvement in survival for treated patients. This improvement is subject to criticism, however, because of several issues, including the fact that it was an unplanned subset analysis [11]. An additional retrospective analysis by Cormier and colleagues [12] basically supports the findings of this meta-analysis. This study analyzed a uniform cohort of AJCC stage III patients from two institutions who were treated from 1984 to 1999 with local therapy only (n = 338) or with local therapy plus DOX (n = 336). DOX was associated with no improvement in disease-specific survival (DSS) [12]. Unfortunately, this study analyzes patients treated over 2 decades, does not perform a contemporary cohort analysis, and does not perform any subset analyses. In addition, important information about the chemotherapeutic regimens employed, specifically the number of patients that received ifosfamide, is not specified.

In the early 1990s, ifosfamide-based chemotherapy (IF) for patients who had primary soft tissue sarcomas was introduced as a promising treatment based on the responses generated in the treatment of metastatic disease [13–15]. The few randomized controlled clinical trials performed using IF have arrived at different conclusions and are limited in

---

* Corresponding author.
E-mail address: fceilber@mednet.ucla.edu (F.C. Eilber).

orthopedic.theclinics.com

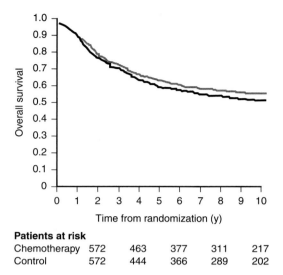

Patients at risk

Chemotherapy	572	463	377	311	217
Control	572	444	366	289	202

Fig. 1. Lancet sarcoma meta-analysis: overall survival for adjuvant DOX versus control. (*From* Adjuvant chemotherapy for localized resectable soft-tissue sarcoma of adults: meta-analysis of individual data. Sarcoma Meta-analysis Collaboration. Lancet 1997;350:1651; with permission.)

their impact because of inclusion of multiple, non-extremity tumor sites; heterogeneity of histologic types; and small sample sizes [16–18]. The most promising of these studies by Frustaci and colleagues [18] demonstrated a significant survival benefit at 4 years in 53 patients treated with IF (Fig. 2). The 5-year overall survival benefit remains statistically

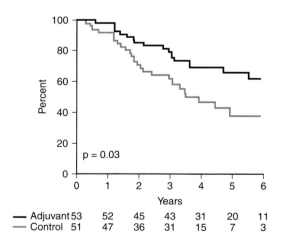

— Adjuvant	53	52	45	43	31	20	11
— Control	51	47	36	31	15	7	3

Fig. 2. Italian Cooperative Trial: overall survival for adjuvant IF versus control. (*From* Frustaci S, Gherlinzoni F, DePaoli A, et al. Adjuvant chemotherapy for adult soft tissue sarcoma of the extremity and girdles: results of the Italian randomized cooperative trial. J Clin Oncol 2001; 19:1244; with permission.)

significant after 7 years of follow-up; however, the overall survival in an intent-to-treat analysis is no longer statistically significant [19]. Additional factors diminishing the impact of this study are that the control no-chemotherapy arm had a much poorer survival than is typically found in patients who have high-risk extremity lesions, and histologic subtype—a prognostic factor for survival—was not stratified for, resulting in an imbalance between the treatment and no-treatment arms. These factors may account for, or at least contribute to, the survival differences demonstrated in this study.

Several recent retrospective analyses have also found that IF is associated with an improved survival in patients who have high-risk primary extremity soft tissue sarcomas [20–22]. Eilber and colleagues [20] found that in 125 patients treated with neoadjuvant, protocol, IF had a significantly increased pathologic response and improved survival compared with patients treated with doxorubicin-based protocols (no ifosfamide) (Fig. 3). However, the protocols compared in this study were performed at different times, and differences in prognostic factors, such as histologic subtypes, were not accounted for. DeLaney and colleagues [21] found that in 48 patients treated with neoadjuvant, protocol chemotherapy containing mesna/doxorubicin/ifosfamide/dacarbazine had a significant reduction in distant metastases and an

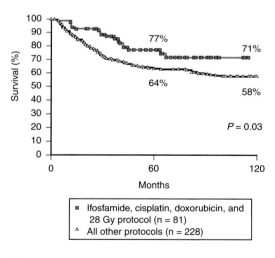

Fig. 3. UCLA neoadjuvant chemotherapy protocol comparison: survival for IF versus DOX (no ifosfamide). Protocol comparison (N = 309) (■, ifosfamide, cisplatin, doxorubicin, and 38 Gy protocol [n = 81]; ▲, all other protocols [n = 228]). (*From* Eilber FC, Rosen G, Eckardt J, et al. Treatment induced pathologic necrosis: a predictor of local recurrence and survival in patients receiving neoadjuvant therapy for high grade extremity soft tissue sarcomas. J Clin Oncol 2001;19:3207; with permission.)

improved disease-free and overall survival compared with a control group. Although the control group was matched for tumor size, grade, age, and era of treatment, it was not matched for histologic subtype, and 12 of the 48 control patients received other chemotherapy regimens. Grobmyer and colleagues [22] analyzed a contemporary cohort of patients from two institutions who were treated from 1990 to 2001 with surgery only (n = 282) or neoadjuvant chemotherapy containing doxorubicin/ifosfamide/mesna (AIM) (n = 74). Adjusting for known prognostic factors, AIM chemotherapy was associated with a significant improvement in disease-specific survival. This improvement was most pronounced in patients who had large tumors. The 3-year DSS for patients who had tumors larger than 10 cm was 62% for patients not treated with chemotherapy and 83% for patients treated with AIM chemotherapy [22].

Although these studies suggest that IF offers a survival benefit to some high-risk patients who have primary extremity soft tissue sarcomas, this benefit may be histology- and size-specific. Unfortunately, it is difficult to identify the benefit to a specific histologic subtype in studies that group all histologies together. The most common histology in the Lancet meta-analysis is "other" (n = 492, 31%) and in the Eilber study is liposarcoma (n = 134, 27%) [10,20]. Malignant fibrous histiocytoma, a historically non-specific diagnosis that has fallen out of favor as a distinct histologic entity [23,24], is the most common histology in the Cormier study (n = 250, 37%), in the Frustaci study (n = 28, 28%), in the DeLaney study (n = 36, 38%), and in the Grobmyer study (n = 201, 56%) [12,18,21,22]. Because of the rarity and diversity of soft tissue sarcomas, no institution has been able to amass an adequate number of high-risk patients at a pace that would permit histology-specific randomized treatment comparisons. Despite this, the value of identifying histology-specific treatment is becoming progressively more important in the current era where soft tissue sarcomas are being classified and treated based on their molecular and genetic characteristics [25].

In attempt to overcome the inherent limitations encountered when studying a rare and histologically diverse malignancy, several investigators have recently begun to analyze the impact of chemotherapy in a histology-specific manner through the use of large sarcoma databases [26–28]. The two studies that merit particular attention used the large, prospectively collected sarcoma databases from two major sarcoma centers: Memorial Sloan-Kettering Cancer Center (MSKCC) and the University of California, Los Angeles (UCLA) [26,27].

Synovial sarcoma

Synovial sarcoma was chosen for analysis for several reasons. It comprises 10% to 15% of adult soft tissue sarcomas. The extremity is the most common site of primary disease [1,8]. It predominately occurs in young adults, is by definition histologically high grade and has been considered to present a poor prognosis when compared with other soft tissue sarcomas [29–33]. Among patients who have primary extremity synovial sarcomas that are 5 cm or larger in size, distant metastases arise in up to 70%, with a resulting 5-year tumor-specific mortality of over 50% [31]. Although IF has been shown to generate impressive responses in the treatment of metastatic and pediatric synovial sarcoma, its impact on the survival of adult patients who have primary disease remains uncertain [34–37]. The objective of the synovial sarcoma study was to determine if IF offered a survival benefit to adult patients who have high-risk primary extremity synovial sarcoma [26].

The prospective sarcoma databases from MSKCC (1982–2002) and UCLA (1975–2002) were used to identify all adult patients (age ≥ 16 years) who had deep primary extremity synovial sarcomas that were 5 cm or larger who underwent surgical treatment for cure (N = 157). The study analyzed the treatments that were administered to the primary tumor, taking into consideration the type of surgical procedure, radiation therapy, and chemotherapy (neoadjuvant or adjuvant). All patients underwent complete surgical resection of their primary tumor at either MSKCC or UCLA. Patients were grouped as having been treated with radiation therapy (external beam radiation or brachytherapy) or not. The type of chemotherapy was grouped into one of three treatment groups: (1) Patients who received no chemotherapy for the primary tumor (NoC), (2) patients who were treated with DOX (defined as patients who were treated with doxorubicin chemotherapy for the primary tumor either alone or in combination with other non–ifosfamide-containing regimens), and (3) patients who were treated with IF (defined as patients who were treated with ifosfamide chemotherapy for the primary tumor either alone or in combination with other agents).

As IF was first used to treat patients in 1990, a contemporary cohort of all patients treated from 1990 to 2002 (N = 103) was used to study the impact of IF on DSS, distant recurrence-free survival (DRFS), and local recurrence-free survival (LRFS). During this period, 33 received NoC, 2 patients were treated with DOX, and 68 patients were treated with IF. The two patients treated with DOX were excluded, resulting in 101 patients for analysis [26]. There was an almost identical number of patients treated at MSKCC (N=50, 50%) and at UCLA (N = 51, 50%). Ninety-four (93%) patients underwent surgical resection of the primary tumor, with seven (7%) requiring amputation. Out of 94 patients, 89 (95%) who underwent limb-sparing surgery received adjuvant radiation therapy and 5 out of 94 (5%) did not. Of the five patients who did not receive radiation therapy, three received NoC and two received treatment with IF.

The clinical, pathologic, and treatment variables of each treatment group were similar [26]. The median tumor size was 7.2 cm (range, 5–25 cm) for the patients treated with IF and 7 cm (range, 5–18 cm) for the patients treated with NoC. The histologic subtypes of the patients treated with IF were 46 (68%) monophasic and 22 (32%) biphasic. The histologic subtypes of the patients treated with NoC were 23 (70%) monophasic and ten (30%) biphasic. The only major difference was institutional treatment. Of the patients treated with IF, 48 (71%) were treated at UCLA and 20 (29%) at MSKCC. Of the patients treated with NoC, 30 (91%) were treated at MSKCC and three (9%) at UCLA.

With a median follow-up of 58 months for survivors, treatment with IF was significantly associated with DSS (P = .01). The 4-year DSS was 88% in patients treated with IF and 67% in patients treated with NoC (Fig. 4). By multivariate analysis, treatment with IF and smaller size were independently associ-

ated with an improved DSS. Patients who did not receive IF had a threefold increased risk of death from disease compared with patients who received IF [26].

Treatment with IF was significantly associated with DRFS (P = .002). The 4-year DRFS of the patients treated with IF was 74% compared with 46% for the patients treated with NoC. As with DSS, treatment with IF and smaller size were independently associated with an improved DRFS [26]. Treatment with IF was not associated with LRFS (P = .39). The 4-year LRFS of the patients treated with IF was 89% compared with 81% for the patients treated with NoC. Multivariate analysis revealed that no variable was associated with an improved LRFS.

The fact that there was a significant improvement in DRFS but not LRFS suggests that the improvement in DSS associated with IF compared with NoC is caused by the treatment of subclinical systemic disease. Whether treatment with IF has completely eliminated subclinical systemic disease (preventing the development of distant recurrences) or whether it has just significantly slowed its growth (delaying the development of distant recurrences) will become more evident with longer follow-up. Regardless, treatment with IF should be strongly considered in patients who have large primary extremity synovial sarcoma.

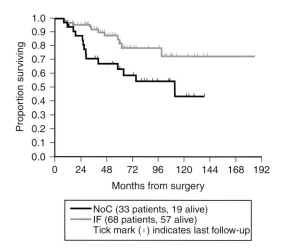

Fig. 4. Synovial sarcoma (1990–2002): disease-specific survival for IF versus no chemotherapy. Tick mark indicates last follow-up. (*Data from* Eilber FC, Eilber FR, Eckardt J, et al. Impact of ifosfamide-based chemotherapy on survival in patients with primary extremity synovial sarcoma [abstract 9017]. Proc Am Soc Clin Oncol 2004;23:818.)

Liposarcoma

As with synovial sarcoma, liposarcoma was chosen for analysis for several straightforward reasons. It is the most common soft tissue sarcoma, with the extremity being the most common site of primary disease [1,8]. In patients who have high-grade extremity liposarcomas that are larger than 5 cm, distant metastasis may occur in 25% of dedifferentiated lesions, in 50% of myxoid/round cell lesions, and in 75% of pleomorphic lesions [38]. The objectives of the liposarcoma study were broader than the synovial analysis, as there were more patients available for analysis. As such, the intent was to determine if any chemotherapy offered a survival benefit to patients who had high-risk primary extremity liposarcoma [27].

All patients who had high-grade, primary extremity liposarcoma (n = 245) of larger than 5 cm were identified from the prospective sarcoma databases at MSKCC (1982–2003) and UCLA (1976–2003). Patients were treated with NoC (n = 99, 40%), DOX (n = 83, 34%), and IF (n = 63, 26%). Although the patients treated with NoC span the entire study period

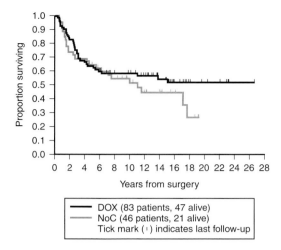

Fig. 5. Liposarcoma (1975–1990): DSS for DOX versus no chemotherapy. Tick mark indicates last follow-up. (*From* Eilber FC, Eilber FR, Eckardt J, et al. The impact of chemotherapy on the survival of patients with high-grade primary extremity liposarcoma. Ann Surg 2004;240(4):689; with permission.)

from 1975 to 2003, the patients treated with DOX were essentially treated in a different decade (1975–1990) from the patients treated with IF (1990–2003). Thus, to accurately assess the impact of treatment with DOX and IF, two separate contemporary cohort analyses were performed [27].

A cohort of patients treated from 1975 to 1990 was used to study the impact of DOX on DSS; 129 patients were identified. Eighty-three (64%) patients received treatment with DOX and 46 (36%) with NoC. There was a similar number of patients treated at MSKCC (N = 62, 48%) and at UCLA (N = 67, 52%). The clinical and pathologic characteristics of the patients treated with DOX were similar to the patients treated with NoC, with the only major difference being institutional treatment. Most patients from UCLA were treated with DOX (n = 62, 75%), and most patients from MSKCC were treated with NoC (n = 41, 89%). With a median follow-up of over 14 years for survivors, treatment with DOX was not significantly associated with DSS (P = .28). The 5-year DSS of the patients who were treated with DOX was 64% compared with 56% for the patients treated with NoC (Fig. 5). Multivariate analysis also revealed that treatment with DOX was not associated with an improved DSS (P=.92) [27].

A cohort of patients treated from 1990 to 2003 was used to analyze the impact of IF on DSS, DRFS, and LRFS; 126 patients were identified. Sixty-three (50%) patients received treatment with IF and

63 (50%) with NoC. There was a similar number of patients treated at MSKCC (N = 62, 49%) and at UCLA (N = 64, 51%). Of these patients, 119 (94%) underwent surgical resection of the primary, with seven (6%) requiring amputation. Of the 119 patients who underwent limb-sparing surgery, 112 (94%) received adjuvant radiation therapy and seven (6%) did not. Of the seven patients who did not receive radiation therapy, four received NoC and three received IF treatment [27].

The clinical and pathologic characteristics of the patients treated with IF were similar to the patients treated with NoC. The median tumor size was 11.5 cm (range, 6–30 cm) for the patients treated with IF and 12 cm (range, 5.2–37 cm) for the patients treated with NoC. For the patients treated with IF, the histologic subtypes were: 31 (49%) myxoid/round cell, 24 (38%) pleomorphic, and eight (13%) dedifferentiated. For the patients treated with NoC, the histologic subtypes were: 30 (48%) myxoid/round cell, 27 (42%) pleomorphic, and six (10%) dedifferentiated. Again, the only major difference between these treatment groups was institutional treatment. Most of the patients from UCLA were treated with IF (n = 55, 87%) and most of the patients from MSKCC were treated with NoC (n = 54, 86%) [27].

With a median follow-up of 60 months for survivors, treatment with IF was found to be significantly associated with DSS (P = .003). The 5-year DSS was 92% in the patients treated with IF and 65% in the patients treated with NoC (Fig. 6). By

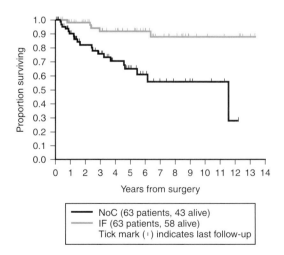

Fig. 6. Liposarcoma (1990–2003): DSS for IF versus no chemotherapy. Tick mark indicates last follow-up. (*From* Eilber FC, Eilber FR, Eckardt J, et al. The impact of chemotherapy on the survival of patients with high-grade primary extremity liposarcoma. Ann Surg 2004;240(4):690; with permission.)

multivariate analysis treatment with IF, myxoid/round cell histologic subtype and smaller size were independently associated with an improved DSS. Patients who did not receive IF had a threefold increased risk of death from disease compared with patients who received IF. In addition, patients who had pleomorphic liposarcoma had a fourfold increased risk of death from disease compared with patients who had the myxoid/round cell subtype.

Additional analyses were performed to determine if there was a tumor size range that benefited most from treatment with IF. Although there was a modest (14%) survival benefit at 5 years for patients treated with IF who had a tumor size of 10 cm or smaller, there was a 31% survival benefit at 5 years for patients treated with IF who had a tumor size larger than 10 cm [27].

As with DSS, treatment with IF was significantly associated with DRFS ($P = .02$). The 5-year DRFS of the patients treated with IF was 81% compared with 63% for the patients treated with NoC. Treatment with IF was not associated with LRFS ($P = .99$). The 5-year LRFS of the patients treated with IF was 86% compared with 87% for the patients treated with NoC [27]. As with synovial sarcoma, the improvement in DSS associated with IF appears to be driven by the treatment of subclinical systemic disease, and treatment with IF should be considered in patients who have high-risk primary extremity liposarcoma.

Synovial sarcoma & liposarcoma UCLA/MSKCC database analyses

The most evident limitation of these studies is that they are retrospective cohort analyses, not randomized trials. Even though the patients from UCLA were treated with neoadjuvant chemotherapy in a protocol manner, the treatments at UCLA and MSKCC were nonrandomized and ultimately administered on the basis of physician judgment, reflecting the evolution of treatment at each institution. The fact that a median of eight patients per year who have two of the most common high-risk primary extremity soft tissue sarcomas are being treated at UCLA and MSKCC combined demonstrates how uncommon these tumors are and how difficult it would be to perform a histology-specific randomized trial in soft tissue sarcomas. Despite this difficulty, it is becoming increasingly important to identify histology-specific treatment in an era where it is being learned how distinct these tumors are [25]. Until multicenter national or international studies are organized to accrue

sufficient numbers of patients to perform histology-specific randomized trials, database analyses from such institutions will provide the best data to estimate survival benefit from systemic treatment.

Although the investigators deliberately placed the focus on ifosfamide by describing the treatment as IF, it is important to recognize that all of these patients were also treated with doxorubicin. Based on the analysis of the evolution of treatment protocols at UCLA, it appears that ifosfamide is responsible for the improvement in survival among these patients [20]. However, the contribution of the individual chemotherapeutic agents or the possible synergy between ifosfamide and doxorubicin cannot be assessed by this study.

In summary, DOX was not associated with an improved DSS compared with patients who had high-risk primary extremity liposarcomas who received no chemotherapy [27]. In patients who have high-risk primary extremity synovial sarcoma and liposarcoma, IF was associated with an improved DSS compared with patients who received no chemotherapy. This improvement in DSS appears to be driven by an improvement in DRFS not LRFS [26,27].

Summary

DOX does not seem to offer a survival benefit to patients who have high-risk primary extremity soft tissue sarcomas, whereas IF does. This benefit is likely histology- and size-specific. Until a less toxic targeted systemic therapy is developed, treatment with IF should be strongly considered in patients who have high-risk primary extremity soft tissue sarcomas.

References

[1] Brennan M, Alektiar KM, Maki RG. Soft tissue sarcoma. In: DeVita VT, Hellmann S, Rosenberg SA, editors. Cancer. Principles and practice of oncology. Philadelphia: Lippincott Williams & Wilkins; 2001. p. 1841–91.

[2] Eilber FC, Eilber FR. Soft tissue sarcoma. In: Cameron JL, editor. Current surgical therapy. 7th edition. St. Louis (MO): Mosby; 2001. p. 1213–8.

[3] American Joint Committee on Cancer. Cancer staging manual. 6th edition. New York: Springer; 2002.

[4] Singer S, Corson JM, Gonin R, et al. Prognostic factors predictive of survival and local recurrence for extremity soft tissue sarcoma. Ann Surg 1994;219:165–73.

[5] Pisters PW, Leung DH, Woodruff J, et al. Analysis of prognostic factors in 1,041 patients with localized soft

tissue sarcomas of the extremities. J Clin Oncol 1996; 14:1679–89.

[6] Coindre JM, Terrier P, Bui NB, et al. Prognostic factors in adult patients with locally controlled soft tissue sarcoma. A study on 546 patients from the French Federation of Cancer Centers Sarcoma Group. J Clin Oncol 1996;4:869–77.

[7] Lewis JJ, Leung D, Casper ES, et al. Multifactorial analysis of long-term follow-up (more than 5 years) of primary extremity sarcoma. Arch Surg 1999;134: 190–4.

[8] Eilber FC, Rosen G, Nelson S, et al. High grade extremity soft tissue sarcomas: Factors predictive of local recurrence and its effect on morbidity and mortality. Ann Surg 2003;237(2):218–26.

[9] Eilber FC, Brennan MF, Riedel E, et al. Prognostic factors for survival in patients with locally recurrent extremity soft tissue sarcomas. Ann Surg Oncol 2005; 12(3):228–36.

[10] Adjuvant chemotherapy for localised resectable soft-tissue sarcoma of adults: meta-analysis of individual data. Sarcoma Meta-analysis Collaboration. Lancet 1997; 350:1647–54.

[11] Verweij J, Seynaeve C. The reason for confining the use of adjuvant chemotherapy in soft tissue sarcoma to the investigational setting. Semin Radiat Oncol 1999; 9(4):352–9.

[12] Cormier JN, Huang X, Xing Y, et al. Cohort analysis of patients with localized, high-risk, extremity soft tissue sarcoma treated at two cancer centers: chemotherapy-associated outcomes. J Clin Oncol 2004; 22(22):4567–74.

[13] Antman KH, Ryan L, Elias A, et al. Response to ifosfamide and mesna: 124 previously treated patients with metastatic or unresectable sarcoma. J Clin Oncol 1989;7(1):126–31.

[14] Antman KH. Chemotherapy of advanced sarcomas of bone and soft tissue. Semin Oncol 1992;19:13–20.

[15] Antman K, Crowley J, Balcerzak SP, et al. An intergroup phase III randomized study of doxorubicin and dacarbazine with or without ifosfamide and mesna in advanced soft tissue and bone sarcomas. J Clin Oncol 1993;11(7):1276–85.

[16] Brodowicz T, Schwameis E, Widder J, et al. Intensified adjuvant IFADIC chemotherapy for adult soft tissue sarcoma: a prospective randomized feasibility trial. Sarcoma 2000;4:151–60.

[17] Gortzak E, Azzarelli A, Buesa J, et al. A randomized phase II study on neo-adjuvant chemotherapy for "high-risk" adult soft-tissue sarcoma. Eur J Cancer 2001;37:1096–103.

[18] Frustaci S, Gherlinzoni F, DePaoli A, et al. Adjuvant chemotherapy for adult soft tissue sarcoma of the extremity and girdles: results of the Italian randomized cooperative trial. J Clin Oncol 2001;19:1238–47.

[19] Frustaci S, De Paoli A, Bidoli E, et al. Ifosfamide in the adjuvant therapy of soft tissue sarcomas. Oncology 2003;65(2):80–4.

[20] Eilber FC, Rosen G, Eckardt J, et al. Treatment in-duced pathologic necrosis: a predictor of local recurrence and survival in patients receiving neoadjuvant therapy for high grade extremity soft tissue sarcomas. J Clin Oncol 2001;19:3203–9.

[21] DeLaney TF, Spiro IJ, Suit HD, et al. Neoadjuvant chemotherapy and radiotherapy for large extremity soft-tissue sarcomas. Int J Radiat Oncol Biol Phys 2003; 56(4):1117–27.

[22] Grobmyer SR, Maki RG, Demetri GD, et al. Neo-adjuvant chemotherapy for primary high grade extremity soft tissue sarcoma. Ann Oncol 2004;15(11): 1667–72.

[23] Fletcher CD, Unni KK, Mertens F. World Health Organization Classification of Tumors. In: Pathology and genetics of tumours of soft tissue and bone. Lyon (France): IARC Press; 2002. p. 120–3.

[24] Fletcher CD. Pleomorphic malignant fibrous histiocytoma: fact or fiction? A critical reappraisal based on 159 tumors diagnosed as pleomorphic sarcoma. Am J Surg Pathol 1992;16:213–28.

[25] Borden EC, Baker LH, Bell RS, et al. Soft tissue sarcomas of adults: state of the translational science. Clin Cancer Res 2003;9(6):1941–56.

[26] Eilber FC, Eilber FR, Eckardt J, et al. Impact of ifosfamide-based chemotherapy on survival in patients with primary extremity synovial sarcoma [abstract 9017]. Proc Am Soc Clin Oncol 2004;23:818.

[27] Eilber FC, Eilber FR, Eckardt J, et al. The impact of chemotherapy on the survival of patients with high-grade primary extremity liposarcoma. Ann Surg 2004; 240(4):686–95.

[28] Ferrari A, Gronchi A, Casanova M, et al. Synovial sarcoma: a retrospective analysis of 271 patients of all ages treated at a single institution. Cancer 2004;101: 627–34.

[29] Hajdu SI, Shiu MH, Fortner JG. Tendosynovial sarcoma: a clinicopathological study of 136 cases. Cancer 1977;39:1201–17.

[30] Singer S, Baldini EH, Demetri GD, et al. Synovial sarcoma: prognostic significance of tumor size, margin of resection and mitotic activity for survival. J Clin Oncol 1996;14:1201–8.

[31] Lewis JJ, Antonescu CR, Leung DH, et al. Synovial sarcoma: a multivariate analysis of prognostic factors in 112 patients with primary localized tumors of the extremity. J Clin Oncol 2000;18:2087–94.

[32] Spillane AJ, A'Hern R, Judson IR, et al. Synovial sarcoma: a clinicopathologic, staging, and prognostic assessment. J Clin Oncol 2000;18:3794–803.

[33] Trassard M, Le Doussal V, Hacene K, et al. Prognostic factors in localized primary synovial sarcoma: a multicenter study of 128 adult patients. J Clin Oncol 2001; 19:525–34.

[34] Rosen G, Forscher C, Lowenbraun S, et al. Synovial sarcoma: Uniform response of metastases to high dose ifosfamide. Cancer 1994;73:2506–11.

[35] Kampe CE, Rosen G, Eilber F, et al. Synovial sarcoma: A study of intensive chemotherapy in 14 patients with localized disease. Cancer 1993;72:2161–9.

[36] Landenstein R, Treuner J, Koscielniak E, et al. Synovial sarcoma of childhood and adolescence: report of the German CWS-81 study. Cancer 1993;71: 3647–55.

[37] Okcu MF, Munsell M, Treuner J, et al. Synovial sarcoma of childhood and adolescence: a multicenter, multivariate analysis of outcome. J Clin Oncol 2003; 21:1602–11.

[38] Dei Tos AP. Liposarcoma: new entities and evolving concepts. Ann Diagn Pathol 2000;4(4):252–66.

Orthop Clin N Am 37 (2006) 23 – 33

Pigmented Villonodular Synovitis

Onder Ofluoglu, MD

Orthopedic Surgery and Trauma Clinic, Lutfi Kirdar Education and Research Hospital, Istanbul, Turkey

Pigmented villonodular synovitis (PVNS) is a rare disease characterized by idiopathic proliferation of synovial tissue in the joint, tendon sheath, and bursa. It appears in two forms: diffuse or localized. When the entire synovium is affected, the condition is referred to as diffuse PVNS (DPVNS). When a single discrete mass is present in the synovium, it is called localized PVNS. Both forms may arise from intra-articular or extra-articular synovial tissues. The term *giant cell tumor of the tendon sheath* is used for tenosynovial involvement. Although histologic and cytogenetic features of these conditions are identical, they present a different clinical course and are regarded as separate entities [1–3].

PVNS is a locally aggressive lesion that may invade and destroy surrounding soft tissue and bone, resulting in functional deterioration of the joint and the extremity. It may involve any synovial joint; however, the large joints are affected frequently. The most common localization of DPVNS is at the knee, followed by the hip, shoulder, and other joints [4]. Involvement of the axial skeleton (mainly in the posterior elements of spine) has been reported, albeit rarely [5,6]. The localized form frequently occurs at the flexor tendon sheaths of the hand and represents the second most common hand tumor following ganglion cysts. The foot is also frequently involved. PVNS affects both sexes equally and occurs at any age, with the greatest incidence in adults in their thirties and forties. It is typically a monoarticular disease; however, a rare polyarticular or multifocal involvement has been reported [7]. Pediatric cases may be associated with a wide range of congenital anomalies [8–10].

PVNS was first described by Chassaignac [11] in 1852 as a nodular lesion arising from the synovial membrane of the flexor tendons of the middle finger. Until 1941, it was considered a benign but sometimes malignant lesion. It was named variably (such as synovial xanthoma, synovial endothelioma, xanthogranuloma, xanthomatous giant cell tumor, myeloplexoma, and fibrohemosideric sarcoma), mostly implying its neoplastic origin. Jaffe and colleagues [12] in 1941 grouped this variety of fibrohistiocytic lesions with the same microscopic appearance under the name PVNS and considered that it was a nonneoplastic inflammatory reaction to an unknown agent or agents.

Etiology

Since the first description of a lesion, there has not been a consensus as to whether its nature is inflammatory or neoplastic in origin. Formerly, localized disturbance of lipid metabolism and recurrent bleeding were frequently considered factors in the etiology of PVNS; however, these ideas were not supported by others. Experimental studies conducted by injection of lipids, blood, or iron failed to produce the lesion, although mild transient alterations were observed [13,14].

Several recent studies based on ultrastructural and cytogenetic analysis suggest that the lesion is a more neoplastic than inflammatory process. Rao and Vigorita [15] proposed distinct differences between the lesion and the adjacent synovial tissue, and centrifugal growth patterns were emphasized to prove

E-mail address: oofluoglu@yahoo.com

doi:10.1016/j.ocl.2005.08.002

that it is a neoplasia. Ultrastructural studies demonstrated that the lesion has two predominate cell types: mononuclear cells that exhibit phenotypic features consistent with derivation from a monocyte/macrophage lineage, and multinuclear cells that are differentiated osteoclastic giant cells from a monocyte [16]. Neale and colleagues [17] also showed that these giant cells expressed osteoclast antigenic phenotype, tartrate-resistant acid phosphatase (a sensitive marker for osteoclasts), and calcitonin receptor (specific marker for osteoclasts) positivity. The close association of the giant cells and osteoclasts was also demonstrated by other studies [18,19]. In addition, there was expression of matrix metalloproteinases (MMP), which are Zn^{2+}-dependent extra-articular enzymes such as collagenase and stromelysin, by synovial lining cells and expression of MMP-2 and MMP-9 by mononuclear and multinuclear cells [20]. These findings suggest that the pathogenesis of the bone erosions/cysts, a consequence of aggressive behavior of the PVNS, might be mediated by osteoclast-like giant cells expressing proteolytic enzymes.

The results of the studies regarding whether PVNS is monoclonal or polyclonal in origin are also controversial. Some studies showed a monoclonal-type cell proliferation, suggesting a neoplastic process of PVNS, whereas others showed a polyclonal origin, supporting a hyperplastic or reactive origin [21–24]. The various numeric and structural chromosomal aberrations in PVNS were described. Of those, trisomy for chromosomes 5 and 7 are the most commonly reported karyotypic abnormalities, although these studies were performed on a limited number of cases and revealed variable results of 0% to 56% in frequency [25,26]. The presence of trisomy 7 in normal synovial fibroblasts and non-tumoral synovial disorders like osteoarthritis, rheumatoid arthritis, and hemorrhagic synovitis suggests that there is uncertainty for correlation between the presence of trisomy and PVNS [27–29].

Another common chromosomal abnormality is the structural rearrangement of chromosome 1, which has been observed in diffuse and localized forms. Sciot and colleagues [3] and Nilsson and coworkers [30] reported that this chromosomal alteration was the most frequent finding, occurring in 58% to 92% of the lesions. Similar changes were noted in only 20% of the investigated cases [25].

Other cytogenetic abnormalities in PVNS are rearrangement of 16q24 and 2q35-37, the gains on chromosomes 16 to 22, and aneuploid DNA pattern [25,30–32]. Despite the growing number of cytogenetic findings, their relevance and significance to the origin of PVNS need to be further studied.

Clinical presentation

The clinical findings of PVNS depend on the location and extent of the disease (Table 1). Onset is insidious and its course shows a slow, progressive character. In the diffuse form, mild pain and limitation of range of motion are the main symptoms. These symptoms are commonly related to joint effusions that show an episodic character—the patient may have completely symptom-free periods between exacerbations. In superficial joints like the knee and the ankle, the swelling and local warmth due to effusion are easily noted. Aspiration of a joint may reveal brown fluid or, more infrequently, characteristic hemarthrosis [33]. A mild contracture or blocking of flexion or extension as a result of synovial hypertrophy may be found. In localized PVNS of the joints, swelling and mechanical symptoms such as locking, giving way, and catching are more prominent [34]. Becasue the symptoms are non-specific and mimic internal derangements or arthritis of the joints, there can be a considerable delay in diagnosis of up to a few years.

Spinal PVNS is a rare condition, with half of the cases localized to the cervical spine and the rest in thoracic and lumber areas. Posterior elements are frequently involved at the affected region. Spinal lesions may be manifested by neurologic symptoms in addition to pain [5,6].

Imaging

A plain radiograph may be normal or may reveal nonspecific changes depending on the severity of the disease. In the knee joint, it shows an increased soft-tissue density at the anterior or posterior synovial sac with or without a lobulated mass, which indicates synovial hypertrophy and joint effusion (Fig. 1). Soft-tissue calcification is an unusual finding. Bony changes including marginal erosions and cysts sur-

Table 1
Clinical presentation of pigmented villonodular synovitis

Form	Tissue
Diffuse	Intra-articular
	Extra-articular (pigmented villonodular bursitis)
	Mixed
Localized	Intra-articular
	Extra-articular (giant cell tumor of the tendon sheaths)

rounded by thin sclerosis occur in one third of the diffuse lesions, particularly in a chronic setting. Although the pathogenesis of these lesions is not known, it is thought that the lesions are a result of increased intra-articular pressure due to the effusion and synovial hypertrophy on the cartilage and underlying bone. Another explanation is direct osseous invasion of the synovium through the vascular foramina along the epiphyseal vessels [35,36]. The former theory may also explain why the bony lesions are seen earlier and more frequently in the hip joint, which has a tight capsule and ligaments without any synovial recesses that limit its capacity to expand [33,35,37]. Osteophyte formation is rare and joint-

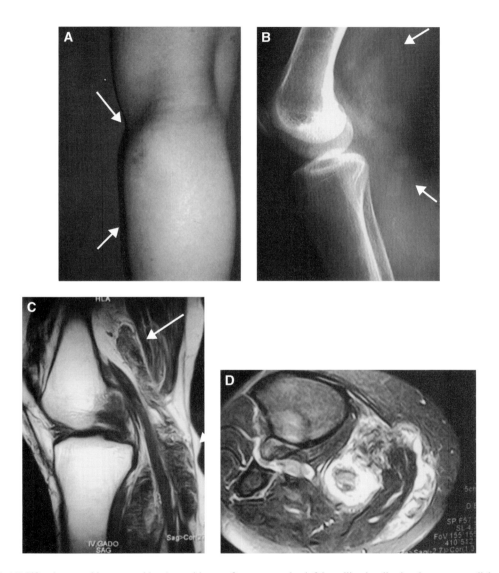

Fig. 1. (A) Fifty-six-year-old woman with a 4-year history of recurrent and painful swelling localized at the posteromedial region of the right knee (arrows). (B) Lateral roentgenogram of the knee shows posteriorly localized lobulated soft tissue mass with increased density (arrows). (C) Sagittal T1-weighted MRI of the knee with contrast shows large soft tissue mass localized at semitendinosus and gastrocnemius bursae associated with posterior involvement of the knee joint adjacent to the posterior cruciate ligament (arrow). (D) Gadolinum-enhanced axial T2-weighted MRI at the level of proximal tibia demonstrates heterogeneous mass surrounding the medial head of the gastrocnemius muscle with strong enhancement. (E) Light-microscopic appearance of the surgical specimen shows mononuclear cells, multinuclear giant cells, lipid-laden macrophages, and hemosiderin deposition surrounded by synovial lining cells (hematoxylin-eosin, original magnification ×40).

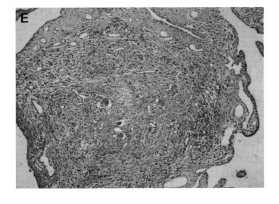

Fig. 1 (*continued*).

space narrowing is usually not seen until late in the disease [38].

Arthrography of the knee may demonstrate a single intra-articular mass in a localized form or multiple nodular or ill-defined filling defects with an enlarged capsule. Ultrasonographic appearance includes a markedly thickened synovium, joint effusion, and heterogeneous echogenic mass reflecting hyperemia. These findings are also seen in intra-articular soft tissue tumors or infectious, inflammatory synovial lesions using both imaging modalities

and therefore considered nondiagnostic for PVNS [33,39]. On CT scans, the increased iron content of synovial tissue appears as a high-density soft tissue mass. Extension of synovial proliferation can be seen effectively with a contrast-enhanced image. CT is particularly useful to demonstrate the bone lesions [40].

Currently, MRI is the preferred imaging modality for PVNS. In addition to diagnosis, it also reveals detailed information regarding the extent of the disease (Fig. 2). The tissue composition of PVNS (including hemosiderin, lipid, and fibrosis) determines the appearance on the MRI. Characteristic findings include hyperplastic synovium with heterogeneous signal intensity in all the imaging sequences as a combination of low signal intensity areas (created by paramagnetic effects of hemosiderin deposits and fibrous tissue) and high signal intensity areas (representing congested synovium and fat content). The low signal blooming effect of hemosiderin is best seen on T2-weighted gradient-echo images. Joint effusion at the periphery of the lesion is noted as low–intermediate signal on proton density T1; high signal on T2-weighted sequences. Contrasted images demonstrate marked enhancement depending on the amount of inflammation and vascularity [2,37,39–41]. This pattern of enhancement may be useful to differentiate the synovium from

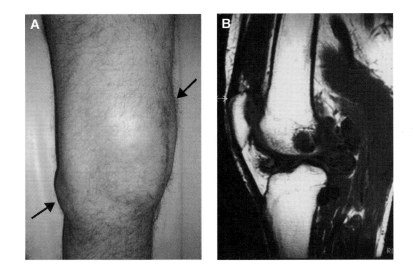

Fig. 2. (*A*) Thirty-nine-year-old man with recurrent DPVNS of the left knee and marked swelling at the suprapatellar and posteromedial area of the joint with scars from previous surgeries (*arrows*). (*B*) T1-weighted sagittal MRI of the knee shows lobulated low signal intensity soft tissue masses at suprapatellar pouch and popliteal fossa with extracapsular extension. A cystic cavity within the medial femoral condyle demonstrated by low signal intensity is also noted. (*C*) T2-weighted gradient-echo coronal section through the suprapatellar pouch shows marked low signal intensity areas. (*D*) Sagittal T1-weighted image and (*E*) T2-weighted image after contrast administration shows marked enhancement as a result of inflammation and vascularity. Extension of the lesion is also seen.

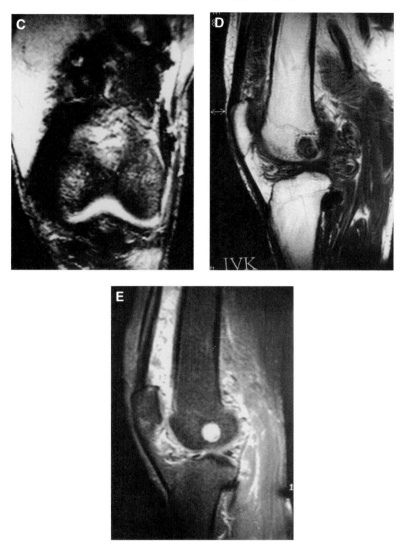

Fig. 2 (*continued*).

the nonenhanced fluid and to help define the extent of the lesion. The cystic bone lesions show a decreased signal compared with surrounding fluid and bone marrow changes, which represent a high signal. Bone lesions are not found in pediatric patients [42].

Differential diagnosis

The differential diagnosis of PVNS includes diseases resulting in synovial hyperplasia and joint destruction including monoarthritis, intra- or juxta- articular synovial tumors, and hemophilia. Biopsy is indicated for suspected lesions (Box 1).

Treatment

Diffuse pigmented villonodular synovitis

Despite its benign nature, PVNS is locally aggressive and supported by the incidence of recurrences and subsequent joint damage. In DPVNS, the recurrence rate is significantly high, as reported in 10% to 56% of cases [12,41,43,44]. The actual rate may

Box 1. Differential diagnosis of diffuse
pigmented villonodular synovitis

Monoarthritis causing
    synovial hypertrophy
  Osteoarthritis
  Rheumatoid arthritis
  Tuberculous arthritis
Synovial tumors
  Synovial hemangioma
  Synovial chondromatosis
  Lipoma arborescens
  Synovial sarcoma
Hemophilic arthropathy

be even higher if MRI is used as a detection method [45].

Recurrence may occur as early as within the first postoperative month or many years after the operation. Schwartz and coworkers [4] reported that the mean time for recurrence was about 5 years and the risk increases with time: 7% at 1 year, 15% at 5 years, and nearly 35% at 25 years. Studies attempting to define factors that contribute to recurrence showed that location (more frequent in knee joint), history of previous operations, and most important, positive surgical margins have predictive value. Other factors are not established with findings of clinical picture such as sex; irradiation; presence of bone cysts; histology such as gross appearance, cellularity, and mitotic index; and cytogenetic findings such as chromosomal abnormalities or the expression pattern of cell cycle–related gene products while comparing primary and recurrent forms [46–48].

Clinical investigations showed that the results of an incomplete synovectomy are associated with a high rate of residual tumor and subsequent recurrences (Table 2).

Byres and colleagues [43] reviewed a series of 24 patients who had DPVNS of the knee joint. Except for 4 cases treated by arthrodesis or amputation, all others were treated by synovectomy. These investigators reported 46% recurrence after synovectomy.

Schwartz and colleagues [4] investigated the treatment results of 99 patients at a mean of 13.5 years follow-up. Seventy-four patients underwent complete or incomplete synovectomy, and synovectomy plus prosthetic replacement was done in the remaining 25. Recurrences were observed in 25 patients after the first procedure. Twenty of 56 patients (35%) showed recurrence in the incomplete synovectomy group, and 5 of 18 patients (27%) showed recurrence in the complete synovectomy group. No recurrences were seen in patients treated with synovectomy plus prosthetic replacement.

Johansson and colleagues [44] treated 18 patients who had DPVNS of the knee. Extensive synovectomy was performed in all patients. Six patients

Table 2
Results of treatment of diffuse pigmented villonodular synovitis

Study	N	Localization (n)	Treatment (n)	Follow-up (mo)	Recurrence (n)
Johansson et al [44]	27	Knee (18) Hip (4) Shoulder (3) Ankle (2)	OTS	94	26
Ogilvie-Harris et al [55]	20	Knee	ATS (11) APS (9)	54	9 55
Flandry et al [49]	23	Knee	OTS	58	8
Zvijac et al [54]	12	Knee	ATS	40.9	17
Blanco et al [68]	22	Knee	APS + EBR	33	14
Chin et al [45]	40	Knee	OTS (5) OTS + IRI (30) OTS + EBR (5)	60	18
Shabat et al [70]	10	Knee (6) Ankle (3) Hip (1)	OPS + IRI	72	10
De Ponti et al [56]	15	Knee	ATS (7) APS (8)	60	20 50

Abbreviations: APS, arthroscopic partial synovectomy; ATS, arthroscopic total synovectomy; EBR, external beam radiation; IRI, intraarticular radiocolloid injection; OPS, open partial synovectomy; OTS, open total synovectomy.

(33%) developed recurrence at an average of 7.8 years of follow-up.

Unsatisfactory results with a high recurrence rate encouraged surgeons to seek more aggressive treatment methods to achieve complete synovectomy for eradication of disease. Flandry and coworkers [49] described the open technique of total synovectomy in the knee joint. Multiple approaches were used to access all the compartments of the knee joint and to carry out a complete synovectomy in 23 patients who had DPVNS (19 primary and 4 recurrent). Additional proximal extensor mechanism realignment was done in 9 patients to compensate for the laxity of the extensor mechanism due to chronic distension of the suprapatellar pouch. Follow-up evaluation was done by patient history, clinical symptoms, and radiographic changes. At an average of 58 months of follow-up, only two recurrences (8%) were reported—the lowest rate in the literature. A significant number of cases developed adhesions that restricted joint motion, requiring early joint manipulation under anesthesia. This study indicated that long-term ankylosis was not a problem with early manipulations. Final outcome was rated as excellent or good in 92% of the patients.

Chin and colleagues [45] reviewed the results of a total synovectomy by way of an initial extensile posterior approach of the knee with release of the medial and lateral heads of the gastrocnemius followed by an anterior arthrotomy. Forty patients who had DPVNS were included, all having been referred after having multiple open or arthroscopic surgical procedures such as arthroscopic synovectomy, open synovectomy, artrhoscopic menisectomy, and so forth. In the postoperative period, a continuous passive motion was used for 3 weeks. Complications were stiffness (3 patients), reflex sympathetic dystrophy (1 patient), and arthritic changes that led to total arthroplasty (4 patients). All patients were screened by MRI in the follow-up period. Recurrence was seen in 7 cases (18%), however 93% of the patients were satisfied with the results of procedure.

The arthroscopic total synovectomy of the knee has a recurrence rate similar to the open technique. Compared with open synovectomy, it has less morbidity and a more rapid recovery period. It is a technically demanding procedure and may be associated with potential complications if the surgeon is not experienced or familiar with the posterior knee anatomy. The standard anterior portals are not effective, whereas the accessory posterior portals are necessary to accomplish total posterior synovectomy. Vascular or neurologic injury may occur during this procedure, especially if there is posterior extra-articular extension of the lesion or fibrosis after irradiation. Open synovectomy should be preferred in such cases [50–52]. Arthroscopic total synovectomy is more difficult in other joints such as the hip and shoulder. In these joints, arthroscopy may be useful as the initial diagnostic tool [53].

Zvijac and colleagues [54] treated 12 patients who had DPVNS of the knee with arthroscopic total synovectomy. Four patients had previous open synovectomies before referral. Two patients (17%) had recurrences, which were identified by MRI findings and clinical symptoms; both of these patients had prior synovectomies.

Ogilvie-Harris and coworkers [55] reported the results of arthroscopic synovectomy in 20 patients. Eleven patients underwent complete synovectomy and 9 underwent partial synovectomy. Although the scores for patient satisfaction were similar in both groups, recurrence was significantly lower in the complete synovectomy group (9%) compared with the incomplete group (56%).

De Ponti et al [56] reported the results of arthroscopic treatment of 19 patients who had PVNS. Fifteen patients who had the diffuse form of the disease underwent partial (8 patients) or total (7 patients) synovectomy. No significant complications related to surgery were encountered, although patients treated with extensive synovectomy showed slower functional recovery. In the partial synovectomy group, 50% of recurrence with obvious clinical symptoms (effusion, pain, and movement impairment) occurred within 2 years. This rate was 20% in the total synovectomy group.

Another treatment modality is radiotherapy. External beam radiation with low to moderate doses as a single agent has been used in the treatment of diffuse PVNS. A good response was reported by some investigators, especially in a subset of patients in the early course of the disease, although the follow-up periods in these studies were short [57,58].

Most researchers agree that radiation should be reserved for recurrent lesions and are aware of local complications, such as postradiation fibrosis, swelling, and healing problems of the wound and risks to bone graft incorporation if it is necessary later [59–63]. Malignant transformation after radiation is a worrisome side effect, especially in young patients. In reports of malignant PVNS cases, there is often a history of radiation [64,65].

In current treatment approaches, radiotherapy is recommended as an adjunct to total synovectomy for preventing recurrences in the presence of residual tumor or as second-stage treatment in recurrent cases. Adjuvant radiotherapy is applied by way of external beam radiation or intra-articular radio-colloid injection.

Ustinova and colleagues [66] reported good results after combined treatment with radiotherapy followed by total synovectomy 3 to 4 weeks later in 24 patients who had DPVNS (10 primary and 14 recurrent). Irradiation was given as a single focal dose of 1.2 to 1.5 Gy, 5 fractions per week; the cumulative focal dose reaching 16 to 20 Gy. These investigators reported only one recurrence and satisfactory functional results in most of the cases.

O'Sullivan and coworkers [67] also used external beam radiation in six primary and eight recurrent cases of DPVNS. All of the cases in this study showed intra-articular involvement with considerable extra-articular extension. In a mean 69 months of follow-up, only one recurrence was reported. Eleven patients had excellent or good function of the affected limb and three had fair function.

Blanco and colleagues [68] used postoperative radiotherapy in primary cases of DPVNS of the knee after arthroscopic partial synovectomy limited to the anterior compartment. Radiotherapy was applied in 17 sessions starting 2 weeks after surgery with a total dose of 26 Gy. These investigators reported 86% satisfactory functional results at an average of 33 months of follow-up. A recurrence rate of 14% after this treatment is comparable with the results of a total surgical synovectomy. A short follow-up period and ultrasonographic detection of recurrences may not reflect the actual recurrence rate in this series.

Intra-articular radiocolloid injections with yttrium 90 or dysprosium 165, which are beta emission colloids with very short half-lives, have been used in primary and recurrent cases [63,69]. Shabat and colleagues [70] reported on 10 patients who had DPVNS treated with a combination of debulking surgery and yttrium 90 injection. Four patients underwent more than one surgical procedure and presented with a local recurrence. Intra-articular injection of yttrium 90 was done 6 to 8 weeks after the last surgery, with dose depending on volume of the joint and body size. Mean follow-up was 6 years, and all patients were followed with imaging studies including CT or MRI at 6-month intervals. Excellent functional results without recurrence or complications were noted in 9 patients (90%).

Results of surgery and adjuvant radiotherapy, however, are not uniformly good. Chin and colleagues [45] reviewed the results of 40 patients who had DPVNS. MRI was used for postoperative follow-up in this study. Except for 5 patients who were treated with surgery alone, all others received radiotherapy (radiation synovectomy with dysprosium 165 in 30 patients and external beam radiation in 5 patients) starting 3 months after surgery. These investigators reported that the recurrence rate was 18% despite adjuvant radiotherapy. Similarly, de Visser and coworkers [71] reported that radiosynovectomy alone or in combination with surgery did not give better results than surgical synovectomy. They treated 29 patients who had DPVNS. Seventeen patients were treated with total or subtotal synovectomy. Radiosynovectomy alone or combination with surgical synovectomy was used in the remaining 12 cases. There were 19 recurrences after the first treatment. After the second treatment, residual tumor was found in 10 cases and the lesion recurred in 1 case. Tumor rests or recurrences were found frequently in radiosynovectomy group, but the functional results were satisfactory in most patients despite a high rate of a residual or recurrent tumor.

Minor complications of radiocolloid injections include febrile reactions, soft tissue radionecrosis, and needle-tract pigmentation, which are regarded as predictable and avoidable. The local or systemic spread of radiocolloids is an important complication that may potentially result in infertility and chromosomal damage, which poses a questionable risk for malignant transformation. The estimated systemic leakage of radioactivity outside the joint is very low. Despite wide use of these agents, including treatment of rheumatoid arthritis, no relationship with a secondary malignancy has been reported so far [70,72].

Total joint arthroplasty or arthrodesis is indicated in patients who develop joint destruction with secondary arthritis [35,44,73,74]. A complete synovectomy is performed before the reconstruction and helped by adequate exposure.

In preparation for the knee arthroplasty, resection of the posterior cruciate ligament aids adequate exposure of the synovium for resection. Joint stiffness may occur in the early postoperative period after total joint arthoplasty, especially in the multiply operated patient. This can be addressed by manipulation under anesthesia or by soft tissue release in resistant cases. Recurrence is still possible after complete synovectomy and joint arthroplasty, having a similar rate to total synovectomy alone. If the components are stable, then the recurrence can be treated with repeated synovectomy or radiotherapy depending the extent of the lesion. Amputations have occasionally been used for uncontrolled disease [41,74].

Localized pigmented villonodular synovitis

In contrast to diffuse lesions, localized PVNS in intra- and extra-articular locations can be treated uneventfully by simple excision. Arthroscopic local excision of intra-articular localized PVNS is uniformly successful, resulting in complete relief of symptoms. Most studies report no evidence of recurrence of the lesion after arthroscopic excision [34,55,56,75,76].

Summary

PVNS is local aggressive disease that affects joints, tendon sheaths, and bursae and characterized by benign synovial proliferation of unknown etiology. It exists in diffuse and local forms and represents intra-articular, extra-articular, or mixed-type involvement. Clinical symptoms in the diffuse form include pain, impairment of movement, and joint effusion that shows recurrences and relapses. The localized form may be manifested by symptoms such as internal derangements of the joint. MRI is very helpful in diagnosis and shows a typical heterogeneous signal appearance (a combination of low signal effect of hemosiderin and fibrosis and high signal effect from inflammation and fat content). Primary cases of DPVNS are treated by complete synovectomy, which can be accomplished by arthroscopic or open techniques if the lesion is located within the joint. In cases of extra-articular involvement, open synovectomy is indicated. Incomplete synovectomy is associated with a high incidence of recurrence. Postoperative radiotherapy with low to moderate doses may be beneficial if there is residual tumor or recurrence. Advanced cases with secondary arthritis should be addressed with arthrodesis or arthroplasty plus extensive synovectomy to decrease recurrence. Localized PVNS can be treated with simple excision using arthroscopic or open surgery.

References

[1] O'Connell JX. Pathology of the synovium. Am J Clin Pathol 2000;114:773–84.

[2] Greenspan A, Remagen W. Tumors and tumor-like lesions of the joints. In: Differential diagnosis of tumors and tumor-like lesions of bones and joints. Philadelphia: Lippincott Raven; 1998. p. 389–422.

[3] Sciot R, Rosai J, Dal Cin P, et al. Analysis of 35 cases of localized and diffuse tenosynovial giant cell tumor: a report from the chromosomes and morphology (CHAMP) study group. Genes Chromosomes Cancer 1993;6(4):212–7.

[4] Schwartz HS, Unni KK, Pritchard DJ. Pigmented villonodular synovitis: a retrospective review of affected large joints. Clin Orthop 1989;247:243–5.

[5] Motamedi K, Murphey MD, Fetsch JF, et al. Villonodular synovitis of the spine. Skeletal Radiol 2005; 34:185–95.

[6] Karnezis TA, McMillan RD, Ciric I. Pigmented villonodular synovitis in a vertebra. J Bone Joint Surg Am 1990;72(6):927–30.

[7] Kay R, Eckardt JJ, Mirra JM. Multifocal pigmented villonodular synovitis in a child. Clin Orthop 1996; 322:194–7.

[8] Lindenbaum BL, Hunt T. An unusual presentation of pigmented villonodular synovitis. Clin Orthop 1977; 122:263–7.

[9] Vedantam R, Strecker WB, Schoenecker PL, et al. Polyarticular pigmented villonodular synovitis in a child. Clin Orthop 1998;348:208–11.

[10] Wagner ML, Spjut HJ, Dutton RV, et al. Polyarticular pigmented villonodular synovitis. AJR Am J Roentgenol 1981;136:821–3.

[11] Chassaignac M. Cancer de la gaine des tendons. Gaz Hop Civ Milit 1852;57:185–6.

[12] Jaffe HL, Lichtenstein L, Sutro CJ. Pigmented villonodular synovitis, bursitis and tenosynovitis. A discussion of synovial and bursal equivalents of tenosynovial lesion commonly denoted as xanthoma, xanthogranuloma, giant cell tumor, or myeloplaxoma of tendon sheath, with some considerations of this tendon sheath lesion itself. Arch Pathol 1941;31:731–65.

[13] Flandry F, Hughston JC. Current concepts review. Pigmented villonodular synovitis. J Bone Joint Surg Am 1987;69(6):942–9.

[14] Granowitz SP, D'Antonio J, Mankin HL. The pathogenesis and long-term end results of pigmented villonodular synovitis. Clin Orthop 1976;114:335–51.

[15] Rao AS, Vigorita VJ. Pigmented villonodular synovitis (giant-cell tumor of the tendon sheath and synovial membrane): a review of eighty-one cases. J Bone Joint Surg Am 1984;66(1):76–94.

[16] Darling JM, Goldring SR, Harada Y, et al. Multinucleated cells in pigmented villonodular synovitis and giant cell tumor of tendon sheath express features of osteoclasts. Am J Pathol 1997;150(4):1383–93.

[17] Neale SD, Kristelly R, Gundle R, et al. Giant cells in pigmented villonodular synovitis express an osteoclast phenotype. J Clin Pathol 1997;50(7):605–8.

[18] Hansen T, Petrow PK, Gaumann A, et al. Expression of cysteine proteinases cathepsins B and K and of cysteine proteinase inhibitor cystatin C in giant cell tumor of tendon sheath. Mod Pathol 2001;14(4):318–24.

[19] Yoshida W, Uzuki M, Kurose A, et al. Cell characterization of mononuclear and giant cells constituting pigmented villonodular synovitis. Hum Pathol 2003; 34(1):65–73.

[20] Darling JM, Glimcher LH, Shortkroff S, et al. Expression of metalloproteinases in pigmented villonodular synovitis. Hum Pathol 1994;25(8):825–30.

[21] Choong PF, Willen H, Nilbert M, et al. Pigmented villonodular synovitis monoclonality and metasta-

ses: a case for neoplastic origin? Acta Orthop Scand 1995;66:64–8.

[22] Ray RA, Morton CC, Lipinski KK, et al. Cytogenetic evidence of clonality in a case of pigmented villonodular synovitis. Cancer 1991;67(1):121–5.

[23] Sakkers RJB, de Jong D, Van der Heul RO. X-chromosome inactivation in patients who have pigmented villonodular synovitis. J Bone Joint Surg Am 1991;73(10):1532–6.

[24] Vogrincic GS, O'Connel JX, Gilks CB. Giant cell tumor of tendon sheath is a polyclonal cellular proliferation. Hum Pathol 1997;28(7):815–9.

[25] Berger I, Rieker R, Ehemann V, et al. Analysis of chromosomal imbalances by comparative genomic hybridization of pigmented villonodular synovitis. Cancer Lett 2005;220:231–6.

[26] Brandal P, Bjerkehagen B, Heim S. Molecular cytogenetic characterization of tenosynovial giant cell tumors. Neoplasia 2004;6(5):578–83.

[27] Dahlen A, Broberg K, Domanski HA, et al. Analysis of the distribution and frequency of trisomy 7 in vivo in synovia from patients with osteoarthritis and pigmented villonodular synovitis. Cancer Genet Cytogenet 2001;131:19–24.

[28] Ecklund E, Broberg K, Westergren-Thorsson G, et al. Proteoglycan production in disomic and trisomy carrying human synovial cells. Matrix Biol 2002;21:325–35.

[29] Mertens F, Orndal C, Mandahl N, et al. Chromosome aberrations in tenosynovial giant cell tumors and nontumorous synovial tissue. Genes Chromosomes Cancer 1993;6(4):212–7.

[30] Nilsson M, Hoglund M, Panagopoulos I, et al. Molecular cytogenetic mapping of recurrent chromosomal breakpoints in tenoynovial giant cell tumors. Virchow Arch 2002;441(5):475–80.

[31] Abdul-Karim FW, El-Naggar AK, Joyce MJ, et al. Diffuse and localized tenosynovial giant cell tumor and pigmented villonodular synovitis: a clinicopathologic and flow cytometric DNA analysis. Hum Pathol 1992;23(7):729–35.

[32] Dal Cin P, Scoit R, De Smet L, et al. A new cytogenetic subgroup in tenosynovial giant cell tumor (nodular synovitis) is characterized by involvement of 16q24. Cancer Genet Cytogenet 1996;87(1):85–7.

[33] Flandry F, Hougston JC, McCann SB, et al. Diagnostic features of diffuse pigmented villonodular synovitis of the knee. Clin Orthop 1994;298:212–20.

[34] Moskovich R, Parisien JS. Localized pigmented villonodular synovitis of the knee. Clin Orthop 1991;271:218–24.

[35] Danzig LA, Gershuni DH, Resnick D. Diagnosis and treatment of diffuse pigmented villonodular synovitis of the hip. Clin Orthop 1982;168:42–7.

[36] Scott PM. Bone lesions in pigmented villonodular synovitis. J Bone Joint Surg Br 1968;50:306–11.

[37] Bhimani MA, Wenz JF, Frassica FJ. Pigmented villonodular synovitis: keys to early diagnosis. Clin Orthop 2001;366:197–202.

[38] Bravo SM, Winalski CS, Weissman BN. Pigmented villonodular synovitis. Radiol Clin N Am 1996;34:311–26.

[39] Masih S, Antebi A. Imaging of pigmented villonodular synovitis. Semin Musculoskelet Radiol 2003;7(3):205–16.

[40] Al-Nakshabandi NA, Ryan AG, Choudur H, et al. Pigmented villonodular synovitis: pictorial review. Clin Radiol 2004;59:414–20.

[41] Della-Valle AG, Piccaluga F, Potter HG, et al. Pigmented villonodular synovitis of the hip. Clin Orthop 2001;388:187–99.

[42] Eckhardt BP, Hernandez RF. Pigmented villonodular synovitis: MR imaging in pediatric patients. Pediatr Radiol 2004;34:943–7.

[43] Byers PD, Cotton RE, Deacon OW, et al. The diagnosis and treatment of pigmented villonodular synovitis. J Bone Joint Surg Br 1968;50:290–305.

[44] Johansson JE, Ajjoub S, Coughlin LP, et al. Pigmented villonodular synovitis of joints. Clin Orthop 1982;163:159–66.

[45] Chin KR, Barr SJ, Winalski C, et al. Treatment of advanced primary and recurrent diffuse pigmented villonodular synovitis of the knee. J Bone Joint Surg Am 2002;84(12):2192–202.

[46] Adem C, Sebo TS, Richle DL, et al. Recurrent and non-recurrent pigmented villonodular synovitis. Ann Pathol 2002;22:448–52.

[47] Somerhausen NSA, Fletcher CDM. Diffuse-type giant cell tumor. Am J Surg Pathol 2000;24(4):479–92.

[48] Weckauf H, Helmchen B, Hinz U, et al. Expression of cell cycle-related gene products indifferent forms of primary versus recurrent PVNS. Cancer Lett 2004;210:111–8.

[49] Flandry FC, Hughston JC, Jacobson KE, et al. Surgical treatment of diffuse pigmented villonodular synovitis of the knee. Clin Orthop 1994;300:183–92.

[50] Chin KR, Brick GW. Extraarticular pigmented villonodular synovitis. Clin Orthop 2002;404:330–8.

[51] Kramer DE, Frassica FJ, Cosgarea AJ. Total arthroscopic synovectomy for pigmented villonodular synovitis of the knee. Techniques Knee Surg 2004;3(1):36–45.

[52] Ogilvie-Harris DJ, Al Thani S. Complications of surgery on synovium and soft tissues. Sports Med Arthrosc Rev 2004;12(3):167–71.

[53] Krebs VE. The role of hip arthroscopy in the treatment of synovial disorders and loose bodies. Clin Orthop 2003;406:48–59.

[54] Zvijac JE, Lau AC, Hechtmann KS, et al. Arthroscopic treatment of pigmented villonodular synovitis of the knee. Arthroscopy 1999;15(6):613–7.

[55] Ogilvie-Harris DJ, McLean J, Zarnett ME. Pigmented villonodular synovitis of the knee. The results of total arthroscopic synovectomy, partial arthroscopic synovectomy and arthroscopic local excision. J Bone Joint Surg Am 1992;74:119–23.

[56] De Ponti A, Sansone V, Malcher MD. Results of arthroscopic treatment of pigmented villonodular synovitis of the knee. Arthroscopy 2003;19:602–7.

[57] Friedman M, Schwartz EE. Irradiation therapy of pigmented villonodular synovitis. Bull Hosp Joint Dis 1957;18:19–32.

[58] Greenfield M, Wallace RM. Pigmented villonodular synovitis. Radiology 1950;54:350–6.

[59] Atmore WG, Dahlin DC, Ghormley RK. Pigmented villonodular synovitis: a clinical and pathological study. Minn Med 1956;39:196–202.

[60] Brien EW, Sacoman DM, Mirra JM. Pigmented villonodular synovitis of the foot and ankle. Foot Ankle Int 2004;25(12):908–13.

[61] Larmon WA. Pigmented villonodular synovitis. Med Clin N Am 1965;49:141–50.

[62] McMaster PE. Pigmented villonodular synovitis with invasion of bone. Report of six cases. J Bone Joint Surg Am 1960;42:1170–83.

[63] Wiss DA. Recurrent villonodular synovitis of the knee. Clin Orthop Relat Res 1982;Sep(169):139–44.

[64] Kalil RK, Unni KK. Malignancy in pigmented villonodular synovitis. Skeletal Radiol 1998;27:392–5.

[65] Layfield LJ, Meloni-Ehrig A, Liu K, et al. Malignant giant cell tumor of synovium (malignant pigmented villonodular synovitis): a histologic and fluorescence in situ hybridization analysis of 2 cases with review of the literature. Arch Pathol Lab Med 2000;124:1636–41.

[66] Ustinova VF, Podliashuk EL, Rodionova SS. Combined treatment of diffuse form of pigmented villonodular synovitis. Med Radiol 1986;31:27–31.

[67] O'Sullivan MM, Yates DB, Pritchard MH. Yttrium 90 synoviectomy—a new treatment for pigmented villonodular synovitis. Br J Rheumotol 1987;26(1):71–2.

[68] Blanco CR, Leon HO, Guthrie TB. Combined partial arthroscopic synovectomy and radiation therapy for diffuse pigmented villonodular synovitis of the knee. Arthroscopy 2001;17(5):527–31.

[69] Franssen MJ, Boerbooms AM, Karthaus RP, et al. Treatment of pigmented villonodular synovitis of the knee with yttrium-90 silicate: prospective evaluations by arthroscopy, histology, and 99mTc pertecnetate uptake measurements. Ann Rheum Dis 1989;48(12):1007–13.

[70] Shabat S, Kollender Y, Merimsky O, et al. The use of surgery and yttrium90 in the management of extensive and diffuse pigmented villonodular synovitis of large joints. Rheumotology 2002;41:1113–8.

[71] De Visser E, Veth RP, Pruszczynski M, et al. Diffuse and localized pigmented villonodular synovitis: evaluation of treatment of 38 patients. Arch Orthop Trauma Surg 1999;119(7–8):401–4.

[72] Sledge CB, Atcher RW, Shortkroff S, et al. Intra-articular radiation synovectomy. Clin Orthop 1984;182:37–40.

[73] Toro FG, Paulos JA, Fuentes DL, et al. Total shoulder arthroplasty in pigmented villonodular synovitis: a case report. J Shoulder Elbow Surg 2002;11(2):188–90.

[74] Hamlin BR, Duffy GP, Trousdale RT, et al. Total knee arthroplasty in patients who have pigmented villonodular synovitis. J Bone Joint Surg Am 1998;80(1):76–82.

[75] Kim SJ, Shin SJ, Choi NH, et al. Arthroscopic treatment for localised pigmented villonodular synovitis of the knee. Clin Orthop 2000;379:224–30.

[76] Perka C, Labs K, Zippel H, et al. Localized pigmented villonodular synovitis of the knee joint: neoplasm or reactive granuloma? A review of 18 cases. Rheumotology 2000;39:172–8.

ORTHOPEDIC
CLINICS
OF NORTH AMERICA

Orthop Clin N Am 37 (2006) 35 – 51

Giant Cell Tumor of Bone

Robert E. Turcotte, MD, FRCSC[a,b,*]

[a]*Division of Orthopaedic Surgery, McGill University, 1650 Cedar Avenue, B5 159.6, Montreal, Quebec, Canada, H3G 1A4*
[b]*Department of Orthopaedic Surgery, McGill University Health Centre, 1650 Cedar Avenue, B5 159.6,*
Montreal, Quebec, Canada, H3G 1A4

Giant cell tumor (GCT) of bone is a benign but locally aggressive tumor that usually involves the end of long bone. Its histogenesis remains unclear. It is characterized by a proliferation of mononuclear stromal cells and the presence of many multinucleated giant cells with homogenous distribution. The name *giant cell tumor* was suggested by Cooper and Travers [1] in 1818. Virchow [2] suggested a malignant potential in 1846. Nélaton [3], a French doctor, was the first to recognize the similarities of the multinucleated giant cell with osteoclasts in 1860. In 1912, Bloodgood [4] reported on the benign nature of GCT. Most of current knowledge of this specific bone tumor has come from Jaffe and colleagues [5].

Clinical history

GCT has a significant incidence, accounting for 20% of all benign bone tumors and 5% of all bone tumors, malignant and benign [6]. Higher incidence has been reported for the Chinese population, in which it can be up to 20% of all bone tumors [7]. Although some series show a slight female predomi-

nance [6,8,9], most support that there is no sex predilection in GCT. GCT of bone most frequently occurs in young adults between 20 and 40 years of age (Fig. 1) [6,9,10]. Occurrence before epiphyseal plate closure is exceptional [6,8,11,122]. GCT can be seen in patients over 50 years old. Although less frequent, this disease needs to be included in the differential diagnosis process of a lytic bone lesion [6,12–17].

Ninety percent of GCT exhibits the typical metaphyseoepiphyseal location. Tumor often extends to the articular subchondral bone or even abuts the cartilage. The joint or its capsule is rarely invaded. In the rare instances in which GCT occurs in a skeletally immature patient, the lesion is likely to be found in the metaphysis [18,19].

The most frequent locations, in decreasing order, are the distal femur, the proximal tibia, the distal radius, and the sacrum (Fig. 2) [6,9,10]. Half of GCTs arise in the knee region. Other frequent sites include the fibular head, the proximal femur, and the proximal humerus. Spine involvement can be seen. The lesion is typically found in the vertebral body and usually spares the posterior elements. It is also eccentric, which is helpful in differentiating it from chordoma [9,20–22] (this is especially true for sacral location). Pelvic GCT is rare [119,120]. Iliac or sacral GCT can cross through the sacroiliac joint to involve the adjacent bone. The tarsal bone is another significant location for GCT, but phalanx, metatarsal, metacarpal, and maxilla are rarely involved. Giant cell reparative granuloma is a frequent tumor in these locations and closely resembles GCT radiographically and histologically. Rare cases of GCT of cranial

* Department of Orthopaedic Surgery, McGill University Health Centre, 1650 Cedar Avenue, B5 159.6, Montreal, Quebec, Canada, H3G 1A4.
E-mail address: robert.turcotte@muhc.mcgill.ca

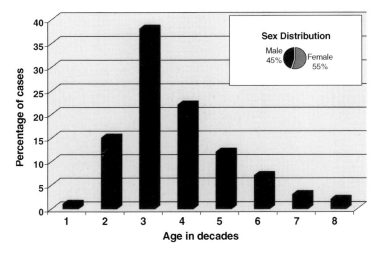

Fig. 1. Age and sex distribution in 1229 cases of GCT of bone from a collection of series by Campanacci [8], Huvos [9], and Unni [6].

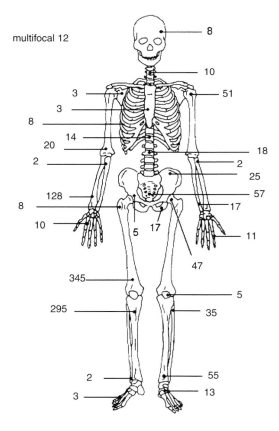

Fig. 2. Anatomic distribution of 1229 GCT of bone from a collection of series by Campanacci [8], Huvos [9], and Unni [6].

bone have been reported and are most often associated with concomitant involvement of the bone by Paget's disease. It is interesting that multiple foci of GCT can be seen within the bone in these instances [13,14,16,25,26]. In addition to this association, multicentricity or the synchronous occurrence of GCT in different bones is known to occur but is exceedingly rare [6,27,28]. Metachronous or sequential occurrence of GTC in different bones is anecdotal but associated with location in the hand or foot when the GCT involves the metaphyseodiaphyseal portion of a long bone. The time interval between the appearance of the first and the subsequent lesions can be many years [29,30]. When facing multicentricity in GCT or if the clinicoradiographic features appear unusual, one should suspect dealing with brown tumor of hyperparathyroidism. Histologically, both lesions are rich in giant cells, which could be confusing. When any clinical doubt exists, patients should be tested for serum calcium, phosphorus, and parathyroid hormone levels.

Pain is the leading symptom in GCT and relates to the mechanical insufficiency resulting from bone destruction, which predisposes patients to fracture. Pathologic fracture is seen in about 12% of patients at the time of diagnosis (Figs. 3A, 4A) [31,32]. A bump or a soft tissue mass can occasionally be seen and results from the cortical destruction and tumor progression outside bone. Because GCT is often found close to the joint, limited range of motion is frequently noticed. Joint effusion and synovitis are also possible. Spinal GCT often has an insidious onset of progressive neck or low back pain. Associated neurologic deficits with these tumors are

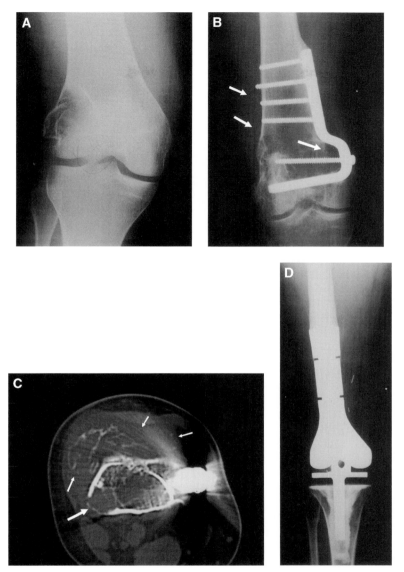

Fig. 3. (*A*) Stage 2 GCT of lateral femoral condyle in a 24-year-old woman showing an intra-articular displaced fracture. Patient was treated in a community hospital with curettage and grafting. A valgus malunion persisted. (*B*) Following bone healing, patient underwent a supracondylar varus osteotomy. Sixteen months following initial surgery, however, she presented with multiple areas of local recurrence (*arrows*). (*C*) CT scan showing areas of recurrence in bone (*large arrow*) and soft tissue (*small arrows*). Note the typical appearance of GCT soft tissue recurrence: nodules devoid of matrix circumscribed by a thin peripheral layer of bone. (*D*) Definitive cure was achieved with a distal femoral replacement showed at 4 years post surgery.

not exceptional, possibly leading to the presumptive diagnosis of disk herniation [26,33–35].

Radiology

Radiographically, GCT of bone displays features that are somewhat characteristic and help in the estab-lishment of a presumptive diagnosis. GCT is usually purely lytic and eccentric within the bone (Fig. 5). As previously stated, in long bones, it is found in the metaphyseoepiphyseal region. The tumor appearance is geographic, with ill-defined borders and often without any identifiable sclerosis. Cortical and can-cellous bone likewise appear destroyed. Although aggressive appearing, a permeative pattern of bone

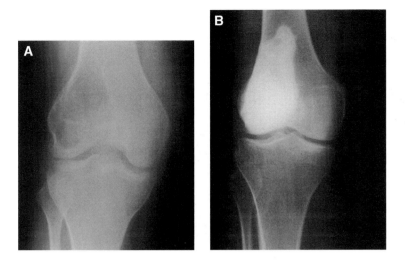

Fig. 4. (*A*) Plain anteroposterior radiograph of the right knee in a 22-year-old woman with a stage 2 GCT complicated by a minimally displaced intra-articular fracture of the lateral femoral condyle. (*B*) Following extended curettage, open reduction and internal fixation was achieved with the use of cement.

destruction is unusual. Bone contour can be expanded with faint and thin periosteal new bone formation. Pseudoseptations are often noted on plain radiographs and are the result of the uneven bone destruction in three dimensions. Tumor matrix is devoid of any ossification or calcification and of similar density to the surrounding soft tissues. CT scan shows the cortical involvement and the soft tissue extension when it exists (Figs. 6B, 7B). The best imaging of full tumor extension is provided, however, by MRI (see Figs. 6C,D and 7C) [36].

Plain radiographs are most helpful in the differential diagnosis that includes GCT. Involvement of the metaphyseoepiphyseal area in a long bone is known to occur most often for three types of bone tumors. GCT is the most frequent, followed by chondroblastoma and, much less frequently, clear cell chondrosarcoma. Chondroblastoma usually occurs in skeletally immature patients. Lesions frequently have a sclerotic rim, and calcifications are seen within the matrix in about 40% [37]. Clear cell chondrosarcoma is found mostly in femoral and humeral heads of young adults. It shows peripheral sclerosis and matrix calcifications and is difficult to distinguish from chondroblastoma before biopsy. Aneurysmal bone cyst (ABC) is another tumor that can look similar to GCT. Although it most often involves the metaphysis of long bone, it is usually devoid of matrix calcifications and peripheral sclerosis. ABC margins are often imprecise, and expansion of the involved bone is usually more marked than in GCT.

GCT, ABC, chondroblastoma, and clear cell chondrosarcoma share the common feature of being eccentric within the bone. Other tumors that should be included in the differential diagnosis are osteosarcoma when it is very lytic or the giant cell–rich variant, malignant fibrous histiocytoma, fibrosarcoma of bone, and plasmocytoma. Metastatic carcinoma should also be considered in the older age group although bone metastases are usually located in the metaphysis or diaphysis of long bones and are less eccentric [38–40].

Similar classifications of GCT based on radiographic appearance were described by Enneking [41] and later by Campanacci [8]. These investigators described three stages that correlate with tumor local aggressiveness and risk of local recurrence. Stage 1 is the least frequent and shows features of latent or slow-growing tumor. The size of the lesion is small, with a mild amount of sclerosis delineating the tumor. Bone contour is not affected, although the cortex can be thinned. The tumor does not extend to the articular cartilage. Symptoms are absent or minimal and of long duration. Stage 2, noted in 75% of GCT at presentation [42], shows features of an active lesion with ill-defined borders and without sclerosis. The cortex is thinned if not breached and deformed with expansion, and the periosteum is elevated. The tumor often extends to the articular cartilage from within the marrow (see Fig. 5). Stage 3 shows extreme aggressiveness, with a tumor of large volume that destroys bone and invades the surrounding soft tissues.

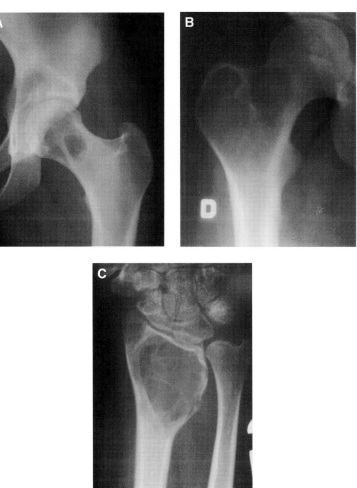

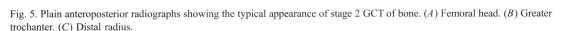

Fig. 5. Plain anteroposterior radiographs showing the typical appearance of stage 2 GCT of bone. (*A*) Femoral head. (*B*) Greater trochanter. (*C*) Distal radius.

Tumor boundaries are imprecise, with possible permeation, which can be suggestive of a malignancy. The tumor abuts the articular cartilage (see Figs. 6 and 7). Tumor growth can be rapid. Higher local recurrence rates are reported with stage 3 tumors and more frequently seen in locally recurrent tumors than in primary presentation (see Fig. 3).

Staging

Although radiographic findings may suggest GCT of bone, as for any suspicious bone lesion, a full staging strategy is highly recommended. This strategy could include a CT scan or MRI of the affected area to evaluate the full local extent of the lesion, a total body bone scan to rule out additional asymptom-

atic bony lesions, and a chest radiograph to exclude lung involvement. Basic blood work can be obtained, although no specific abnormalities are expected. If hypercalcemia and or hypophosphatemia were recorded, then brown tumor and hyperparathyroidism should be high on the differential diagnosis. A biopsy is mandatory to confirm the diagnosis and can be achieved with a core-needle or open biopsy. Principles of musculoskeletal tumor biopsy should be adhered to and (1) include a direct approach in line with the projected incision if a resection is to be performed following the discovery of malignancy; (2) should be vertical, muscle splitting; and (3) the bone window should be oval and good hemostasis should be achieved before wound closure. In centers that have a special interest in bone tumors, the biopsy is often set up to be followed immediately with

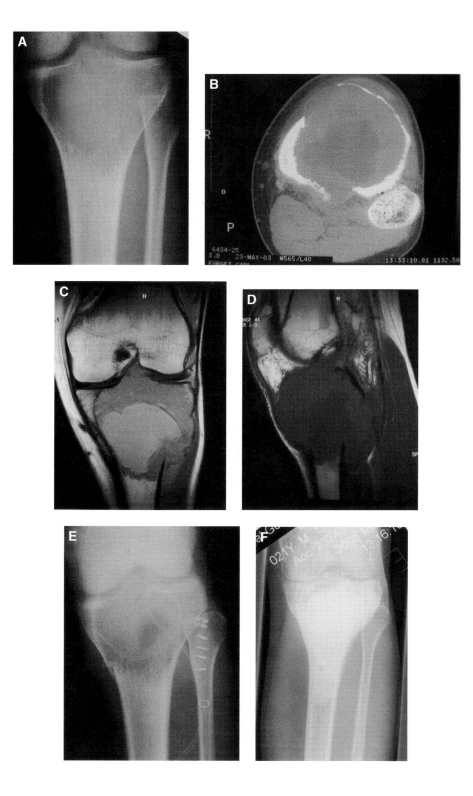

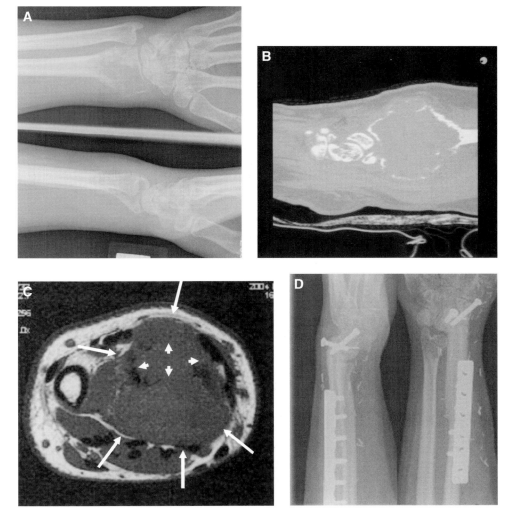

Fig. 7. (*A*) Anteroposterior (*top*) and lateral (*bottom*) plain radiographs of a 20-year-old woman with a stage 3 GCT of distal radius. (*B*) CT scan of sagittal reconstruction showing subchondral bone erosion, deformation, and soft-tissue extension. (*C*) Axial MRI cut shows remains of the original outline of distal radius (*arrowheads*) and extensive soft tissue involvement (*long arrows*). (*D*) Lateral (*left*) and anteroposterior (*right*) radiographs showing results of en bloc resection and reconstruction that used a vascularized fibula to achieve fusion to the proximal carpal row.

curettage if frozen sections confirm the diagnosis of a benign GCT. Interpretation of frozen sections can only be done safely if an experienced bone tumor pathologist is available and good communication exists between the surgeon, the radiologist, and the pathologist. When frozen pathology findings are un-

usual or not in keeping with the radiologic findings (even if it most likely resembles GCT on radiographs), surgery should be delayed until final pathology is available.

At the time of surgery, the cortex is often thinned and perforated in areas. The periosteum can be intact

Fig. 6. Plain radiograph (*A*), CT scan (*B*), and MRI (*C*,*D*) showing a large stage 3 GCT of proximal tibia in a 20-year-old man. (*E*) Open biopsy was complicated by pathologic fracture and became infected. These complications precluded the initial treatment plan of proximal tibial resection and reconstruction with an osteoarticular allograft. (*F*) Packing with antibiotic-loaded cement was performed after extended curettage. Patient has good function 15 months post surgery without evidence of recurrence of infection or tumor.

except in those cases (stage 3) in which it may be absent and the tumor extends into the surrounding soft tissues. Tumor margins are usually well defined in the medullary canal, and small pockets of tumor can be found in cancellous bone with extensions from the main cavity that can easily be overlooked and lead to recurrence. Satellite lesions are rarely expected.

The tumor typically appears red-brown on gross examination. GCT is very vascularized, and hemorragic changes and lipidic degeneration can be encountered. Invasion of ligaments by the tumor is possible. Articular cartilage is usually preserved, even if the subchondral bone has disappeared, and extra care must be taken during curettage. Intra-articular extension of GCT remains exceptional, even in cases of pathologic fracture.

Histology

GCT shows increased cellularity, with numerous multinucleated giant cells uniformly dispersed among a large population of mononuclear cells that are important for diagnosis (Fig. 8). There is little or no intercellular substrate other than a few collagen fibers. Mononuclear cells can be round, oval, polygonal, and sometimes spindled. They exhibit little cytoplasm. The nuclei contain one or more nucleoli and can exhibit variable amounts of hyperchromasia that is different from malignancy. Mitotic figures can be numerous but devoid of abnormalities. The multinucleated cell population exhibits a large volume and their centered nuclei may contain more than a hundred nuclei. These nuclei closely resemble the nuclei of the mononuclear cells. The cytoplasm of the giant cell is

abundant and can contain vacuoles. Numerous blood vessels and capillaries are found, as are areas of necrosis. Reactive bone trabeculae can be seen but is usually at the periphery of the tumor. Intravascular invasion by GCT cells is frequent and more likely seen at the periphery of the lesion. It does not correlate with the incidence of metastasis. Areas of ABC can occur in association with GCT and are seen as blood-filled cavities devoid of endothelial cells.

On histology, the differential diagnosis must include giant cell reparative granuloma and brown tumor of hyperparathyroidism. Both show a more fibrous stroma with multinucleated giant cells containing less nuclei and having a more irregular distribution than in GCT. ABC also shows a smaller number of multinucleated cells with a more fibrous stroma but, strikingly, contains large areas of vascular cavities devoid of endothelial cell lining. Areas of ABC changes can often be identified in GCT. Large sampling is necessary, along with careful review of the radiographs, to make sure that one is not dealing with GCT or other tumors known to be associated with ABC changes when a diagnosis of ABC is made on histology. Giant cell–rich osteosarcoma is a rare variant of osteosarcoma. As its name implies, it shows a large number of multinucleated cells. Its striking feature is the presence of small, malignant, mononuclear cells exhibiting significant atypia and the production of malignant osteoid, albeit often in minimal quantity [6].

Historically, GCT was graded in three histologic grades that are now of little use because they do not correlate with prognosis [8,9]. Giant cell sarcoma is a very rare primary tumor, most frequently associated with recurrence of tumor or following irradiation. Sufficient biopsy sampling is necessary in GCT because sarcomatous areas may exist throughout areas of a benign-looking lesion.

Basic sciences

There is evidence that three types of cells are found in benign GCT of bone [43]. Type I cells look like interstitial fibroblasts, make collagen, and have the capacity to proliferate. This cell population is likely the tumor component of GCT [43]. Type I cells share some features of mesenchymal stem cells from which they could be derived; however, they possess features that suggest they could represent an early differentiation of mesenchymal stem cells into osteoblasts [28,44–46,123]. Type II cells are also interstitial but resemble the monocyte/macrophage family and could be recruited from the peripheral

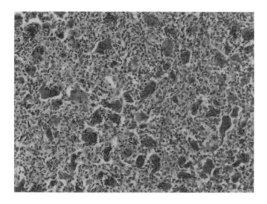

Fig. 8. Typical histologic appearance of benign GCT showing hypercellularity with a population of mononuclear cells and numerous giant multinucleated cells uniformly dispersed.

blood stream [47]. These cells are thought to be precursors of the multinucleated giant cells (by fusing together or by nuclear multiplication without cell division). Type II cells express surface receptors of the monocyte/macrophage lineage but these receptors are not found on giant cells [43]. Type III cells are the multinucleated giant cells. They share many characteristics of osteoclasts and have similar morphologies [48]. They possess enzymes for bone resorption, including tartrate resistant acid phosphatase and type II carbonic anhydrase [49]. GCT giant cells exhibit most of the specific osteoclast antigens [50,51]. Cell receptors for calcitonin and vitronectin are present [43], and expression of matrix metalloproteinases (MMPs) is found [52].

Significant-level activity for insulin-like growth factor I and II is found in type II and type III cells but absent in type I cells, which suggests that these factors are important in the development and regulation of GCT [53]. In addition, it is known that insulin growth factor I plays a role in the formation of osteoclasts from monocytes, augments osteoclast level of activity [54,55], and increases bone resorption [56,57]. Transforming growth factor (TGF)-β1, found in all three cell populations of GCT, is thought to be implicated in the recruitment of the multinucleated cells or their precursors. TGF-β2 is found only in multinucleated cells [58]. MMPs (MMP-9 and MMP-2) are enzymes that act on extracellular matrix and collagen degradation. Tissue inhibitors of metalloproteinases, such as TIMP-1, regulate their activities. MMP and protease activity increases in GCT as the radiographic grade or clinical aggressiveness (such as lung metastases) increases [39,59]. MMP-9 is mostly found in the multinucleated giant cells [52,60,121]. Cathepsin K is also only found in the multinucleated giant cell population [60]. These findings suggest that bone resorption in GCT is achieved through the action of the osteoclast-like giant cells. No specific translocation or chromosomal anomalies are found in GCT, but normal karyotype is rarely encountered. Telomeric fusion, or fusion of two chromosomes by their ends, is a frequent finding compared with other solid tumors. It most often involves chromosome 11. A higher incidence of chromosomic anomalies has been reported for recurrent benign GCT or GCT that metastasizes to lung (97%) than for GCT cured after initial surgery [10].

Treatment

GCT of bone is benign and most frequently involves the end of a long bone adjacent to a joint in a young adult. The best treatment should insure local control and maintain function. Curettage has been the preferred treatment for most cases of GCT. Historically, local recurrence rates of 25% to 50% have been reported (see Figs. 6 and 8) [6–8,13, 14,16,19,61–64]. The most recent series that have included modern imaging techniques and extended curettage through the use of power burrs report improved local recurrence rates (10%–20%) [23, 65–67]. In due consideration, it is preferable to have a conservative approach because most patients can be cured with such curettages, even if reoperation is required.

The recommended curettage technique involves the opening of the bone through a large cortical window that allows visualization of the entire tumor cavity. The use of a headlamp and dental mirrors allows vision of areas difficult to reach directly. Curettes of different sizes allow for curettage of the cavity and the smaller pockets of tumor. After curettage is achieved, the cavity is deepened with the use of high-speed burrs.

Various investigators have proposed the use of local adjuvants in an attempt to achieve a local recurrence rate less than 20% [25,42,63,68]. Phenol [11,22,68,69], liquid nitrogen [70,71], bone cement [62,63,68,72], hydrogen peroxide [21], zinc chloride [73], and more recently, argon beam cauterization have been employed. Chemical or physical agents work by inducing an additional circumferential area of necrosis to "extend" the curettage. Antineoplastic agents such as methotrexate or adriamycin have been studied in addition to cement [74,75]. No clear evidence exists as to whether adjuvants are effective [76], but from retrospective studies, liquid nitrogen has achieved the highest cure rates. Safe handling of liquid nitrogen is difficult, and significant fracture rates have been reported [70,71]. Although the usefulness of bone cement as an adjuvant has recently been questioned [23,64–67,77], there are many advantages to support its use as a cavity filler: (1) it provides immediate mechanical stability, allowing for early weight bearing; (2) it allows for early detection of recurrence [78,79]; and (3) it may have a cytotoxic effect on tumor cells (usually at the cement–bone interface) through the methylmetacrylate monomer and the energy dissipated as the cement sets (cement can induce heat necrosis a few millimeter deep in adjacent bone) [80,81]. Although it appears that cement may be tolerable just underneath the joint surface (Fig. 9C) [82,83], reports have suggested that cement should not be placed deep into the exposed cartilage. Interposing a centimeter or two of bone graft between the cartilage and the cement may

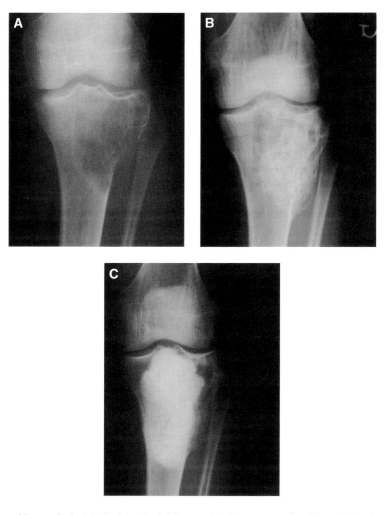

Fig. 9. (*A*) A 25-year-old man who had GCT of proximal tibia treated with curettage and grafting. (*B*) Twelve months later, local recurrence becomes visible on the medial side and under the tibial spines. It is not always easy to detect recurrence with plain radiographs early on because of the bony changes associated with previous treatment and healing. (*C*) Anteroposterior plain radiograph 10 years after additional curettage and cementing.

reduce heat damage and the resultant early degenerative changes [8,84]. Nonetheless, studies have shown that cement constructs are less rigid than normal subchondral bone or successful bone graft [85,86]. In cases of pathologic fracture, cement can also be used to provide a solution to maintain reduction and stability in the fractured eggshell-like cavity (see Fig. 4) [31].

Most recurrent tumors can be treated like primary ones, with extended curettage and grafting or cementing (see Fig. 9) [61,68]. For extensive recurrences, sometimes a sarcoma-like wide resection and reconstruction is indicated (see Fig. 3). The incidence of soft tissue recurrence has been reported to be about

1% [87]. It characteristically appears as a growing nodule, with an incomplete peripheral rim of bone and a center devoid of specific matrix (see Fig. 3C) [8,87,88]. The same phenomenon is sometimes seen with lung metastases from benign GCT. It is strange that these recurrent tumors do not show osteoid above production bone within the lesion. TGF-β1 and TGF-β2 are known to be present in GCT and are involved in the differentiation into osteoblasts of mesenchymal cells originating from adjacent tissue. These TGFs could be responsible for peripheral bone production [88]. It is interesting that intra-articular recurrence of GCT appears to be exceedingly rare, if it ever occurs, even following pathologic fracture.

Wide en bloc resection is known to provide the lowest recurrence rate [25,42,61,89]. This practice is often debatable in the context of benign tumor [67] but can be considered in expendable bones such as the fibula or clavicle. Many stage 3 tumors are treated with such resections, as are multiple local recurrences or pathologic fracture when joint anatomy cannot be restored (see Figs. 3 and 7) [67]. Wide resections/reconstructions can affect function permanently; their results are difficult to compare with conservative surgery because the indications are usually different [61,67]. Reconstruction is achieved as in bone sarcomas, with the use of fibular transfer [90], allograft, endoprosthesis, or arthrodesis (see Figs. 3, 6, and 7); amputation is rarely considered. A more aggressive surgical approach has been recommended by some investigators for GCT arising in the distal radius because local control is more difficult to achieve in this location [23]. Others disagree with this approach and believe that the radius should be treated like any other long bone [67,91]. For large proximal tumors or for difficult locations such as the pelvis, sacrum, and spine, it is wise to proceed with preoperative embolization to minimize bleeding, which can be significant. Embolization may also be attempted to limit progression of an inoperable recurrent tumor. This method of treatment has been reported following repeated embolizations in difficult locations such as the sacrum [92].

Radiotherapy has been used to treat GCT [3,35, 93–95]. It is useful especially in difficult locations such as the spine and sacrum. It has also been advocated to decrease local recurrence. The long-term risk of malignant GCT or postradiation sarcoma has limited its routine use [8,35]. The commonly used dosage is 40 to 45 Gy because total dosage beyond 50 Gy has been associated with a higher risk of malignancy. Use of megavoltage instead of orthovoltage has been reported to not induce sarcomatous changes [95,96]. No formal criteria exist to measure response of GCT to radiation; however, improvement of symptoms, decrease in pain, and progressive ossification suggest a favorable response.

Most local recurrences occur between 12 and 18 months after surgery and rarely after 3 years [8,67]. Local recurrence should be suspected when a progressive area of radiolucency appears within or adjacent to the previously treated area. These areas are more identifiable on plain radiographs when cement has been used as a filler than when bone grafts are used (bone graft healing shows sclerotic and lytic areas; lysis is due to graft resorption) (see Fig. 9). Symptoms appear later as the tumor reaches a significant size. Repeated curettage, even in a multiply recurrent lesion, allows for cure in 80% to 90% of GCT cases without the need for resection. Recurrence rates are still 5% to 10% following resection.

Biphosphonates are drugs that inhibit bone resorption by the osteoclasts. Recent evidence suggests that these agents may have an effect on the giant cell population of GCT by inducing apoptosis and possibly limiting tumor progression [20,97,98]. If confirmed with in vivo and clinical studies, then biphosphonates may offer a novel solution in the treatment of benign GCT of bone and the rare but difficult to treat lung metastases.

Function

Long-term functional results are usually very good after the treatment of GCT, even after curettage and grafting or cementing [66,67]. Pathologic fracture through a GCT may be associated with persistent pain and lowered functional scores.

Lung metastasis from histologically benign giant cell tumor

Although it may seem odd to link lung metastases, a behavior usually associated with malignancy, to a benign bone process, it has been observed by many investigators [17,77,99–107]. The estimated incidence of this phenomenon is 3% [63]. On histology, the lung metastases are identical to benign GCT of bone. Increased incidence of lung metastases is associated with location of primary tumor in the distal radius or sacrum, stage 3 lesions, and multiple local recurrences [16,35,63,77,100]. Dissemination appears to be hematogenous and could happen during curettage, but this remains unproved [9]. Multiple chest nodules, a rare phenomena, may be present but must be confirmed histologically, which can be performed through transthoracic needle biopsy or thoracoscopy or thoracotomy. The latter technique is usually preferred because it allows for full tissue sampling and complete removal of lesions when feasible. If sarcomatous, then this should raise the suspicion that the primary bone tumor was malignant.

It is difficult to predict the behavior of these metastatic benign lesions of the lungs. Spontaneous regression and disappearance have been reported [77]. Progression is usually slow. Reports have suggested up to 70% survival following aggressive

management of lung metastases with repeated surgery [45,77]. For this reason, it is usually wise to
resect them early when possible. In cases in which
lung lesions are unresectable or rapidly recurrent or
multiple, chemotherapy (including interferon) [108]
or radiotherapy could be an option, but their usefulness remains to be confirmed [100,109]. Medi-
astinal lymph node involvement has been reported,
and treatment should be the same as for lung nodules [110].

It is clear that current histologic classification
cannot identify benign-looking GCT that has a more
malignant behavior. In the near future, molecular

biology may lead to a new classification of GCT that
will allow clinicians to tailor treatment modalities and
follow-up studies according to the specific risk of
each tumor.

Malignant giant cell tumors

Malignant GCT or giant cell sarcoma is rare
[24,111–116]. Large series report an incidence of
5%. Spontaneous primary malignant GCT seems exceptional. Malignancy showing as a recurrence of
a previously benign GCT is occasionally seen fol-

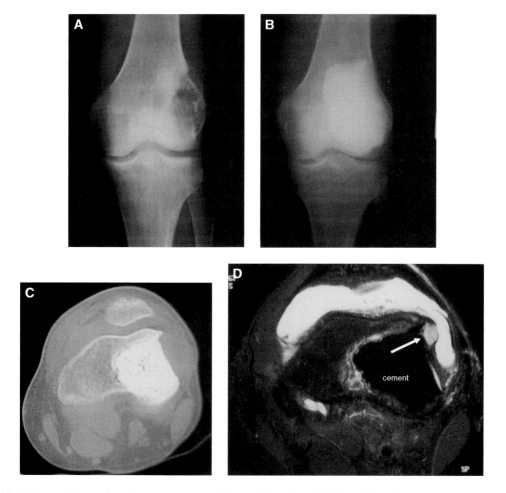

Fig. 10. A 54-year-old man who underwent curettage and autografting of a GCT of lateral femoral condyle in 1969. (*A*) Patient
became symptomatic in 2001 3 months before this plain radiograph was taken. Although suspected, malignant recurrence could
not be diagnosed on histology even after additional outside consultation. (*B*) Anteroposterior plain radiograph following
extended curettage and cementation. (*C*) CT scan and (*D*) MRI showing local recurrence (*arrow*) at periphery of cement
12 months after initial treatment, this time found malignant on histologic sections. (*E*) Treatment included neoadjuvant
chemotherapy and distal femoral resection. Metastatic chest nodules developed 9 months later and were resected. Patient is
currently free of disease 1 year post thoracotomy.

lowing curettage and without previous use of radiation (Fig. 10). The most often encountered scenario is a recurrent malignancy 1 to 10 years or more after irradiation of a previously benign GCT. A dosage as low as 40 Gy could trigger this transformation. This dosage is less than 50 Gy, which is usually recognized to be sufficient to induce postradiation sarcoma, and suggests that benign GCT cells might be prone to malignant transformation. The term *malignant GCT* is controversial because some investigators use it only when there is coexistence within the lesion of areas typical of benign GCT with other areas of frank malignancy changes [117]. It is looked at as areas of dedifferentiation and named according to the morphology of dedifferentiated tissue such as osteosarcoma, malignant fibrous histiocytoma, or fibrosarcoma [118–123]. Malignant GCT is treated like sarcoma (with neoadjuvant chemotherapy and wide resection), achieving a cure rate of 75%. Lung metastasis remains problematic and is addressed with chemotherapy and thoracotomy.

Follow-up

Due to the high incidence of local recurrence and the risk of lung metastasis, a close follow-up of patients who have GCT of bone is required. Follow-up appointments after treatment should be every 3 or 4 months and should include physical examination and plain radiographs of the involved bone. This follow-up allows for early detection of any recurrence. CT scan or MRI can be of great help when

recurrence is suspected. It is unclear whether these imaging modalities have any role for routine follow-up evaluation. Follow-up can be extended to every 6 months after 2 or 3 years. Yearly visits after 5 years up to year 10 are usually recommended. There are no clear recommendations regarding chest surveillance. Chest radiographs should probably be done at every clinic visit. Although a CT scan of the chest may allow for earlier detection of nodules, the low incidence of lung metastasis precludes its routine use. CT scans may be preferred initially, at time of diagnosis, as part of the staging process.

Summary

GCT of bone is a lesion with unpredictable behavior. It presents as a lytic defect in the end of long bone, most frequently affecting the knee area. Although benign, it is locally aggressive and deserves specific treatments that result in decreased local recurrence and preservation of function. Extended curettage followed by cement or bone grafting of some kind is the most often used treatment. En bloc resection is rarely a necessity and is used for more aggressive lesions when the bone or joint surface cannot be salvaged. With modern staging and treatment, the overall local recurrence rate is between 10% and 20%. Local recurrences are usually treated in the same manner as primary tumors. Lung metastasis from benign GCT of bone exists and should be treated vigorously. Malignancy is rarely associated with GCT but may be found in a recurrent tumor (suggesting an initial wrong diagnosis) or years after irradiation of a previously benign GCT. Malignant tumors should be managed in the same manner as sarcomas.

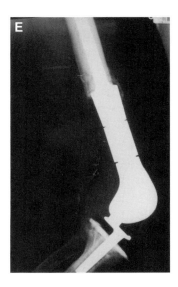

Fig. 10 (*continued*).

References

[1] Cooper AP, Travers B. Surgical essays, vol. I. London: Cot and Son and Longman & Co.; 1818.

[2] Virchow R. Die Krankhaften Geschwulste, vol. 2. Berlin: Hirschwald; 1846.

[3] Nélaton E. D'une nouvelle espèce de tumeur bénigne des os ou tumeur à myéloplaxes. Paris: Adrien Delahaye; 1860.

[4] Bloodgood JC. A conservative treament of giant cell sarcoma with the study of bone transplantation. Ann Surg 1912;56:210–39.

[5] Jaffe HL, Lichtenstein L, Portis RB. Giant cell tumor of bone. Its pathologic appearance, grading, supposed variants and treatment. Arch Pathol 1940;30: 993–1031.

[6] Unni KK. Dahlin's bone tumors: general aspect

and data on 11087 cases. 5th edition. Philadelphia: Lippincott-Raven; 1998.

[7] Sung HW, Kuo DP, Shu WP, et al. Giant cell tumor of bone: analysis of two hundred and eight cases in Chinese patients. J Bone Joint Surg Am 1982;64: 755–61.

[8] Campanacci M. Giant cell tumor. In: Gaggi A, editor. Bone and soft-tissue tumors. Bologna, Italy: Springer-Verlag; 1990. p. 117–53.

[9] Huvos AG. Bone tumors: diagnosis, treatment and prognosis. 2nd edition. Philadelphia: WB Saunders Co.; 1991.

[10] Bridge JA, Neff JR, Mouron BJ. Giant cell tumor of bone: chromosomal analysis of 48 specimens and review of the literature. Cancer Genet Cytogenet 1992;58:2–13.

[11] Picci P, Manfrini M, Zucchi V, et al. Giant cell tumor of bone in skeletally immature patients. J Bone Joint Surg Am 1983;65:486–90.

[12] Carrasco CH, Murray JA. Giant cell tumors. Orthop Clin North Am 1989;20:395–405.

[13] Dahlin DC, Cupps R, Johnson EW. Giant cell tumor: a study of 195 cases. Cancer 1970;25:1061–70.

[14] Eckardt JJ, Grogan TJ. Giant cell tumor of bone. Clin Orthop 1986;204:45–58.

[15] Enneking WF. Musculoskeletal tumor surgery. New York: Churchill-Livingstone; 1983.

[16] Goldenberg R, Campbell CJ, Bonfiglio M. Giant cell tumor of bone. An analysis of two-hundred and eighteen cases. J Bone Joint Surg Am 1970;52: 619–64.

[17] Wilner D. Radiology of bone tumors and allied disorders. Philadelphia: WB Saunders Co.; 1982.

[18] Hoeffel JC, Galloy MA, Grignon Y, et al. Giant-cell tumor of bone in children and adolescents. Rev Rhum 1996;63(9):618–23.

[19] Shih HN, Hsu RW, Sim FH. Excision curettage and allografting of giant cell tumours. World J Surg 1998;22:432–7.

[20] Cheng YY, Huang L, Kumta SM, et al. Cytochemical and ultrastructural changes in the osteoclast-like giant cells of giant cell tumor of bone following biphosphonate administration. Ultrastruct Pathol 2003;27(6): 385–91.

[21] Nicholson NC, Ramp WK, Kneisl JS, et al. Hydrogen peroxide inhibits giant cell tumor and osteoblast metabolism in vitro. Clin Orthop 1998;347:250–60.

[22] Oda Y, Tsuneyoshi M, Iwamoto Y. Giant cell tumour of bone: oncological and functional results of long term follow-up. Jpn J Clin Oncol 1998;28:323–8.

[23] O'Donnel RJ, Springfield DS, Motwani HK, et al. Recurrence of giant cell tumors after curettage and packing with cement. J Bone Joint Surg Am 1994; 76(2):1827–33.

[24] Schajowicz F. Tumors and tumorlike lesions of bone and joints. New York: Springer-Verlag; 1981.

[25] Campanacci M, Baldini N, Boriani S, et al. Giant-cell tumor of bone. J Bone Joint Surg Am 1987;69: 105–44.

[26] Larsson SW, Lorentzon R, Boquist L. Giant-cell tumors of the spine and sacrum causing neurological symptoms. Clin Orthop 1975;111:201–11.

[27] Tornberg D, Dick H, Johnston A. Multicentric giant-cell tumors in the long bones. A case report. J Bone Joint Surg Am 1975;57:420–2.

[28] Wüllling M, Delling G, Kaiser E. The origin of the neoplastic stromal cell in giant cell tumor of bone. Hum Pathol 2003;34(10):983–93.

[29] Cummins CA, Scarborough MT, Enneking WF. Multicentric giant cell tumor of bone. Clin Orthop 1996;322:245–52.

[30] Sybrandy S, De la Fuente AA. Multiple giant-cell tumors of bone. Report of a case. J Bone Joint Surg Br 1973;55:350–6.

[31] Dreinhofer KE, Rydholm A, Bauer HC, et al. Giant cell tumours with fracture at diagnosis. Curettage and acrylic cementing in 10 cases. J Bone Joint Surg Br 1995;77(2):189–93.

[32] Miller G, Bettelli G, Fabbri N, et al. Curettage of giant cell tumor of bone: introduction, material and method. Chir Organi Mov 1990;75(Suppl 1):203–4.

[33] Dahlin DC. Giant cell tumor of vertebrae above the sacrum. A review of 31 cases. Cancer 1977;39: 1350–6.

[34] Turcotte R, Biagini R, Sim FH, et al. Giant cell tumor of the spine and sacrum. Chir Organi Mov 1990;75(Suppl 1):104–7.

[35] Turcotte RE, Sim FH, Unni KK. Giant cell tumor of the sacrum. Clin Orthop 1993;291:215–21.

[36] Hermman SD, Mesgarzadhe M, Bonakdarpour A, et al. The role of magnetic resonance imaging in giant cell tumor of bone. Skeletal Radiol 1987;16:635–43.

[37] Turcotte RE, Kurt A-M, Sim FH, et al. Chondroblastoma. Hum Pathol 1993;24(9):944–9.

[38] Oyasu R, Battifora HA, Buckingham WB, et al. Metaplastic spquamous cell carcinoma of bronchus simulating giant cell tumor of bone. Cancer 1977;39: 1119–28.

[39] Rosai J. Carcinoma of pancreas simulating giant cell tumor of bone. Electron-microscopic evidence of its acinar cell origin. Cancer 1968;22:333–4.

[40] Silverberg SG, De Giorgi LA. Osteoclastoma like giant cell tumor of the thyroid. Cancer 1963;31: 621–5.

[41] Enneking WF. Giant cell tumor. In: Musculoskeletal tumor surgery. New York: Churchill-Livingstone; 1983. p. 1435–68.

[42] Campanacci M, Giunti A, Olmi R. Giant-cell tumors of bone. A study of 209 cases with long-term follow-up in 130. Ital J Orthop Traum 1975;1:153–80.

[43] Goldring SR, Schiller AL, Mankin HJ, et al. Characterization of cells from human giant cell tumors of bone. Clin Orthop 1986;204:59–75.

[44] Huang L, Teng XY, Cheng YY, et al. Expression of proosteoblast markers and Cbfa-1 and Osterix gene transcripts in stromal tumor cells of giant cell tumour of bone. Bone 2004;34(3):393–401.

[45] James IE, Dodds RA, Olivera DL, et al. Human

osteoclastoma-derived stromal cells: correlation of the ability to form mineralized nodules in vitro with formation of bone in vivo. J Bone Miner Res 1996; 11(10):1453–60.

[46] Wüllling M, Delling G, Kaiser E. Differential gene expression in stromal cells of human giant cell tumor of bone. Virchows Arch 2004;445(6):621–30.

[47] Liao TS, Yergulun MB, Cgang SS, et al. Recruitment of osteoclast precursors by stroma cell derived factor-1 (SDF-1) in giant cell tumor of bone. J Orthop Res 2005;23(1):203–9.

[48] Hanaoka H, Friedman B, Mack RP. Ultrastructure and histogenesis of giant cell tumour of bone. Cancer 1970;25:1408–23.

[49] Yoshida H, Akeho H, Yumoto T. Giant cell tumour of bone: histochemical, biochemical and tissue culture studies. Virchows Arch A 1982;395:319–30.

[50] Horton MA, Lewis D, McNulty K, et al. Monoclonal antibodies to osteoclastomas (giant cell bone tumours): definition of osteoclast-specific cellular antigens. Cancer Res 1985;45:5663–9.

[51] James IE, Walsh S, Dodds RA, et al. Production and characterization of osteoclast-selective monoclonal antibodies that distinguish between multinucleated cells derived from different human tissues. J Histochem Cystochem 1991;39:905–14.

[52] Ueda Y, Imai K, Tsuchiya H, et al. Matrix metalloproteinase 9 (gelatinase B) is expressed in multinucleated giant cells of human giant cell tumor of bone and is associated with vascular invasion. Am J Pathol 1996;148(2):611–22.

[53] Middleton J, Arnott N, Walsh S, et al. The expression of mRNA for insulin-like growth factors and their receptor in giant cell tumors of human bone. Clin Orthop 1996;322:224–31.

[54] Mochizuki H, Hakeda Y, Wakatsuki N, et al. Insulin-like growth factor-I supports formation and activation of osteoclasts. Endocrinology 1992;131:1075–80.

[55] Slootweg MC, Most WW, Van Beek E, et al. Osteoclast formation together with interleukin-6 production in mouse long bones is increased by insulin-like growth factor-I. J Endocrinol 1992;132: 433–8.

[56] Ibbotson KJ, Orcutt CM, D'Souza SM, et al. Contrasting effects of parathyroid hormone and insulin-like growth factor I in an aged ovariectomized rat model of postmenopausal osteoporosis. J Bone Miner Res 1992;7:425–32.

[57] Johansson AG, Lindh E, Ljunghall S. Insulin-like growth factor-I stimulates bone turnover in osteoporosis. Lancet 1992;339:1619.

[58] Zheng MH, Fan Y, Wysocki SJ, et al. Gene expression of transforming growth factor-b1 and its type II receptor in giant cell tumors of bone: possible involvement in osteoclast-like cell migration. Am J Pathol 1994;145(5):1095–104.

[59] Gamberi G, Benassi MS, Gagazzini P, et al. Proteases and interleukin-6 gene analysis in 92 giant cell tumors of bone. Ann Oncol 2004;15(3):498–503.

[60] Lindeman JH, Hanemaaijer R, Mulder A, et al. Cathepsin K is the principal protease in giant cell tumor of bone. Am J Pathol 2004;165(2):593–600.

[61] Liu HS, Wang JW. Treatment of giant cell tumor of bone: a comparaison of local curettage and wide resection. Chang Keng I Hsuey 1998;21: 37–43.

[62] Persson BM, Ekelund L, Lövdahl R, et al. Favorable results of acrylic cementation for giant cell tumors. Acta Orthop Scand 1984;55:209–14.

[63] Rock MG. Curettage of giant-cell tumor of bone: factor influencing local recurrences and metastasis. Chir Organi Mov 1990;75(Suppl 1):204–5.

[64] Trieb K, Bitzan P, Dominkus M, et al. Giant-cell tumors of long bone. J Bone Joint Surg Am 2000; 82:1360–1.

[65] Blackley HH, Wunder JS, Davis AM, et al. Treatment of giant-cell tumors of long bone with curettage and bone-grafting. J Bone Joint Surg Am 1999;81:811–20.

[66] Saiz P, Virkus W, Piasecki P, et al. Results of giant cell tumor of bone treated with intralesional excision. Clin Orthop 2004;424:221–6.

[67] Turcotte RE, Davis AM, Wunder J, et al. Giant cell tumour of long bone: a Canadian Sarcoma Group Study. Clin Orthop Rel Res 2002;397:248–58.

[68] Campanna R, Fabbri N, Bettelli G. Curettage of giant cell tumor of bone: the effect of surgical technique and adjuvants on local recurrence rate. Chir Organi Mov 1990;75(Suppl 1):206.

[69] Quint U, Mueller RT, Muller G. Charactheristic of phenol: instillation in intralesional tumor excision of chondroblastoma, osteclastoma and enchondroma. Arch Orthop Trauma Surg 1998;117:43–6.

[70] Malawer MM, Bickels J, Meller I, et al. Cryosurgery in the treament of giant cell tumor: a long term follow-up study. Clin Orthop 1999;359:176–88.

[71] Marcove RC, Weis LD, Vaghaiwalla MR, et al. Cryo-surgery in the tratment of giant cell tumors of bone. A report of 52 consecutive cases. Cancer 1978; 41:957–69.

[72] Bini SA, Gill K, O'Johnston J. Giant cell tumor of bone: curettage and cement reconstruction. Clin Orthop 1995;321:245–50.

[73] Zhen W, Yaotian H, Songjian L, et al. Giant-cell tumour of bone. The long-term results of treatment by curettage and bone graft. J Bone Joint Surg Br 2004;86(2):212–6.

[74] Kirchen ME, Menendez LR, Lee JH, et al. Methtrexate eluted from bone cement: effect on giant cell tumor of bone in vitro. Clin Orthop 1996;328: 294–303.

[75] Zhang Y, Hou C, Chen A. A preliminary observation of giant cell tumor of bone treated by adriamycin-loaded chitosan drug delivery system. Chung Kuo Hsiu Fu Chung Chien Wai Ko Tsa Chih 1998;12: 280–2.

[76] Trieb K, Bitzan P, Lang S, et al. Recurrence of curetted and bone-grafted giant-cell tumours with and

without adjuvant phenol therapy. Eur J Surg Oncol 2001;27(2):200 – 2.

[77] Siebenrock KA, Unni KK, Rock MG. Giant-cell tumor of bone metastasing to the lung: a long term follow-up. J Bone Joint Surg Br 1998;80:43 – 7.

[78] Petterson H, Rydhol A, Persson B. Early detection of local recurrence after curettage and acrylic cementation of giant cell tumors. Eur J Radiol 1986;6:1 – 4.

[79] Remedios D, Saifuddin A, Pringle J. Radiological and clinical recurrence of giant cell tumour of bone after the use of cement. J Bone Joint Surg Br 1997;79:26 – 30.

[80] Mjoberg B, Pettersson H, Rosenqvist R, et al. Bone cement, thermal injury and the radiolucent zone. Acta Othop Scand 1984;55:597 – 600.

[81] Nelson DA, Barker ME, Hamlin BH. Thermal effect of acrylic cementation at bone tumour sites. Int J Hyperthermia 1997;13:287 – 306.

[82] Lavoie S, Turcotte RE, Berthiaume MJ, et al. The arthrogenic effect of cementation for the treatment of giant cell tumor of the knee. J Bone Joint Surg Br 1998;80(Suppl 1):14.

[83] Segura J, Albareda J, Bueno AL, et al. The treatment of giant cell tumors by curettage and filling with acrylic cement. Long term functional results. Chir Organi Mov 1997;82:373 – 80.

[84] Campanacci M, Campanna R, Fabbri N, et al. Curettage of giant cell tumor of bone. Reconstruction with subchondral grafts and cement. Chir Organi Mov 1990;75(Suppl 1):212 – 3.

[85] Frassica FJ, Gorski JP, Sim FH, et al. A comparative analysis of subchondral replacement with polymethylmethacrylate or autogenous bone grafts in dogs. Clin Orthop 1993;293:378 – 90.

[86] Frassica FJ, Sim FH, Pritchard DJ, et al. Subchondral replacement: a comparative analysis of reconstruction with methylmethacrylate or autogenous bone graft. Chir Organi Mov 1990;75(Suppl 1):189 – 90.

[87] Cooper KL, Beabout JW, Dahlin DC. Giant cell tumor: ossification in soft-tissue implants. Radiology 1984;153:597 – 602.

[88] Teot LA, O'Keefe RJ, Rosier RN, et al. Extraosseous primary and recurrent giant cell tumors: transforming growth factor-b1 and -b2 expression may explain metaplastic bone formation. Hum Pathol 1996;27(7):625 – 32.

[89] Campbell CJ, Akbarnia NA. Giant cell tumor of the radius treated by massive resection and tibial bone graft. J Bone Joint Surg Am 1975;57:982 – 6.

[90] Lackman RD, McDonald DJ, Beckenbaugh RD, et al. Fibular reconstruction for giant cell tumor of the distal radius. Clin Orthop 1987;218:232 – 8.

[91] Khan MT, Gray JM, Carter SR, et al. Management of the giant-cell tumours of the distal radius. Ann R Coll Surg Engl 2004;86(1):18 – 24.

[92] Lackman RD, Khoury LD, Esmail A, et al. The treatment of sacral giant-cell tumours by serial arterial embolisation. J Bone Joint Surg Br 2002;84(6):873 – 7.

[93] Caudell JJ, Ballo MT, Zagars GK, et al. Radiotherapy in the management of giant cell tumor of bone. Int J Radiat Oncol Biol Phys 2003;57(1):158 – 65.

[94] Feigenberg SJ, Marcus Jr RB, Zlotecki RA, et al. Radiation therapy for giant cell tumors of bone. Clin Orthop Relat Res 2003;411:207 – 16.

[95] Malone S, O'Sullivan B, Catton C, et al. Long term follow-up of efficacy and safety of megavoltage radiotherapy in high-risk giant cell tumour of bone. Int J Radiat Oncol Biol Phys 1995;33:689 – 94.

[96] Nair MK, Jyothirmayi R. Radiation therapy in the treatment of giant cell tumor of bone. Int J Radiat Oncol Biol Phys 1999;43(5):1065 – 9.

[97] Chang SS, Suratwala SJ, Jung KM, et al. Biphosphonates may reduce recurrence in giant cell tumor by inducing apoptosis. Clin Orthop Relat Res 2004;426:103 – 9.

[98] Cheng YY, Huang L, Lee KM, et al. Biphosphonates induce apoptosis of stromal tumor cells in giant cell tumor of bone. Cal Tissue Int 2004;75(1):71 – 7.

[99] Bertolini F, Present D, Enneking WF. Giant cell tumor of bone with pulmonary metastases. J Bone Joint Surg Am 1985;67:890 – 900.

[100] Bertoni F, Present D, Sudanese A, et al. Giant-cell tumor of bone with pulmonary metastases. Six cases reports and a review of the literature. Clin Orthop 1988;237:275 – 85.

[101] Jewell JH, Bush LF. Benign giant-cell tumor of bone with a solitary pulmonary metastasis. A case report. J Bone Joint Surg Am 1964;46:848 – 52.

[102] Ladanyi M, Traganos F, Huvos AG. Benign metastazing giant cell tumors of bone: a DNA flow cytometric study. Cancer 1998;64:1521 – 6.

[103] Maloney WG, Vaughan LM, Jones HH, et al. Benign metastasizing giant-cell tumor of bone. Report of three cases and review of the literature. Clin Orthop 1983;243:208 – 15.

[104] Pan P, Dahlin DC, Lipscomb PR, et al. Benign giant cell tumor of the radius with pulmonary metastasis. Mayo Clin Proc 1964;39:344 – 9.

[105] Rock MG, Sim FH, Unni KK. Metastases from histologically benign giant-cell tumor of bone. J Bone Joint Surg Am 1984;66:269 – 74.

[106] Vanel D, Contesso G, Rebibo G, et al. Benign giant cell tumors of bone with pulmonary metastases and favorable prognosis. Report in 2 cases and review of the literature. Skeletal Radiol 1983;10:221 – 6.

[107] Wray CC, McDonald AQ, Richardson RA. Benign giant cell tumour with metastases to bone and lung. J Bone Joint Surg Br 1990;72:486 – 9.

[108] Kaiser U, Neumann K, Havemann K. Generalised giant-cell tumour of bone: successful treatment of pulmonary metastases with interferon alpha, a case report. J Cancer Res Clin Oncol 1993;119(5):301 – 3.

[109] Feigenberg SJ, Marcus Jr RB, Zlotecki RA, et al. Whole-lung radiotherapy for giant cell tumors of bone with pulmonary metastases. Clin Orthop Relat Res 2002;401:202 – 8.

[110] Connell D, Munk PL, Lee MJ, et al. Giant cell tumor of bone with selective metastases to mediatinal lymph nodes. Skeletal Radiol 1998;27:341–5.

[111] Boriani S, Sudanese A, Baldani N, et al. Sarcomatous degeneration of giant cell tumors. Ital J Orthop Traum 1986;12:191–9.

[112] Campbell CJ, Bonfiglio M. Aggressiveness and malignancy in giant-cell tumors of bone. In: Price CHG, Ross FGM, editors. Bone: certain aspects of neoplasia. London: Butterworths; 1973.

[113] Gitelis S, Wang J, Quast M, et al. Recurrence of a giant-cell tumor with malignant transformation to a fibrosarcoma twenty-five years after primary treatment. J Bone Joint Surg Am 1990;71:757–61.

[114] Kossey P, Cervenansky J. Malignant giant-cell tumours of bone. In: Price CHG, Ross FGM, editors. Bone: certain aspects of neoplasia. London: Butterworths; 1973.

[115] Murphy WR, Ackerman LV. Benign and malignant giant-cell tumors of bone. A clinical-pathological evaluation of thirty-one cases. Cancer 1956;9:317–39.

[116] Nascimento AG, Huvos AG, Marcove RC. Primary malignant giant cell tumor of bone. A study of eight cases and review of the literature. Cancer 1979;44:1393–404.

[117] Rock MG, Sim FH, Unni KK, et al. Secondary malignant giant cell tumor of bone: clinicopathological assessment of nineteen patients. J Bone Joint Surg Am 1986;68:1073–9.

[118] Meis JM, Dorfman HD, Nathanson SD, et al. Primary malignant giant cell tumor of bone: "dedifferentiated" giant cell tumor. Mod Pathol 1989;2:541–6.

[119] Osaka S, Toriyama S. Surgical treatment of giant cell tumor of the pelvis. Clin Orthop 1987;222:123–31.

[120] Sanjay BKS, Frassica FJ, Frassica DA, et al. Treatment of giant-cell tumor of the pelvis. J Bone Joint Surg Am 1993;75:1466–75.

[121] Schoedel KE, Greco MA, Stetler-Stevenson WG, et al. Expression of metalloproteinases and tissue inhibitors of metalloproteinases in giant cell tumor of bone: an histochemical study with clinical correlation. Hum Pathol 1996;27(11):1144–8.

[122] Sherman M, Fabricius R. Giant-cell tumor in the metaphysis in a child. Report of an unusual case. J Bone Joint Surg Am 1961;43:1225–9.

[123] Wülling M, Engels C, Jesse N, et al. The nature of giant cell tumor of bone. J Cancer Clin Oncol 2001;127:467–74.

ELSEVIER
SAUNDERS

Orthop Clin N Am 37 (2006) 53 – 63

ORTHOPEDIC
CLINICS
OF NORTH AMERICA

Desmoid Tumors and Current Status of Management

Harish S. Hosalkar, MD, MBMS[a], Edward J. Fox, MD[a],*,
Thomas Delaney, MD[b], Jesse T. Torbert, MD[a],
Christian M. Ogilvie, MD[a], Richard D. Lackman, MD[a]

[a]Department of Orthopedic Oncology, University of Pennsylvania, 301 S. 8th Street, Garfield Duncan Bldg.,
Suite 2C, Philadelphia, PA 19106, USA
[b]Department of Medical Oncology, Massachusetts General Hospital, Northeast Proton Therapy Center, 30 Fruit Street,
Boston, MA 02114, USA

Desmoid tumors, also known as aggressive fibromatosis, are rare fibroblastic tumors that exhibit a wide range of local aggressiveness, from largely indolent to locally destructive. Somatic mutations, somatic allele loss, trisomy, and translocation have been demonstrated in these lesions with recent cytogenetic studies, thus conclusively proving them to be true neoplasms. Although these tumors do not have the capacity to metastasize, they can cause extensive morbidity by local destruction of growth patterns and, in some cases, even lead to death.

Understanding of the pathogenesis and the great heterogeneity in the natural history of desmoid tumors is invaluable to the development of therapeutic strategies. The optimal treatment protocol has not yet been established and, in many cases, a multidisciplinary approach including surgery, chemotherapy, and radiation therapy has been employed. The rarity of cases in even major tumor centers has traditionally limited the ability to study this disease. Several novel pharmacologic and biologic treatment approaches are actively being developed, although long-term follow-up is needed for their substantiation.

History and epidemiology

Desmoid tumors account for about 0.03% of all neoplasms and less than 3% of all soft tissue tumors [1]. They were first described in 1832 by MacFarlane [2] of the Royal Glasgow Infirmary [3]. The term *desmoid* originates from the Greek word "desmos," meaning band or tendon-like, and was first applied by Muller [4] to describe tumors with a tendon-like consistency [3].

It remains a rare tumor, with only an estimated 900 new cases diagnosed each year in the United States, or 3 to 4 cases per 1 million people. Desmoids are tumors that occur between the ages of 15 to 60 years, more often in young adulthood, with the median age of diagnosis in the early 30s. There is a twofold to threefold predominance of these lesions in women in most published series [3].

Desmoids occur more commonly in familial adenomatous polyposis (FAP) patients and have a reported incidence of 3.5% to 32% in these patients [5–7]. Metastases have been rarely reported, and progressive sarcomatous transformation is extremely rare. As noted by Hayry and colleagues [8], the only malignant mark of this tumor is its propensity for recurrence and local invasiveness. As such, desmoids continue to present a problem in recognition and management, especially because of the striking discrepancy between its deceptively harmless histologic appearance and its

* Corresponding author.
  E-mail address: edward.fox@uphs.upenn.edu (E.J. Fox).

0030-5898/06/$ – see front matter © 2005 Elsevier Inc. All rights reserved.
doi:10.1016/j.ocl.2005.08.004

propensity toward local recurrence and infiltration of the surrounding soft tissues.

Etiology

The etiology is still an enigma, but desmoids appear to involve a deregulation of connective tissue growth, and the biologic potential of each tumor lesion varies [9]. It is difficult to define the risk factors, considering the rarity and heterogeneity of growth patterns in these lesions. Alman and colleagues [9] identified an abnormal expression of c-sis and platelet-derived growth factor and proposed a mechanism by which inappropriate expression of c-sis can lead to increased production of platelet-derived growth factor, which in turn acts as a mitogen for fibrocytes.

The strongest predisposing factor is the diagnosis of FAP and, more specifically, Gardner's syndrome, a variant of FAP. Almost all patients who have Gardner's syndrome ultimately exhibit malignant transformation of one or more of the polyps. Desmoid tumors occur in approximately 10% of FAP patients or one third of Gardner's syndrome patients [5,6].

FAP and Gardner's syndrome share mutations at chromosome 5q21-22, the locus for the adenomatous polyposis coli (APC) gene [10]. Recent studies have demonstrated that about 15% of desmoids harbor somatic mutations in the APC gene, whose function is to regulate the cellular level of a protein called β-catenin [11,12]. β-catenin acts to alter nuclear transcription and is an important mediator in a signaling system termed Wnt in humans that is important in normal development. These APC mutations in desmoids are considered to cause an increase in β-catenin level, which increases tumor proliferation. All cases of desmoids contain an elevated level of β-catenin level compared with normal cells, regardless of the APC mutations [11]. Thus, β-catenin level may be the underlying cause of the proliferative advantage held by the tumor cells [13]. Transgenic mice expressing a mutant, stabilized β-catenin by way of a tetracycline-driven promoter were found to exhibit increased proliferation, motility, and invasiveness in their fibroblasts with stabilized β-catenin expression. These cells developed into tumors after inoculation into nude mice. β-catenin is a particularly difficult molecule to characterize because of its integral function in multiple diverse cellular activities. Whether this will become a point for targeted therapy in the future remains to be seen [3]. Matrix metalloproteinase activity has recently been noted to modulate tumor size, cell motility, and cell invasiveness in murine aggressive fibromatosis, suggesting that

the efficacy of tissue inhibitors of matrix metalloproteinases [TIMP] might be worth studying in this disease [14].

Predilection for desmoid tumors in Gardner's syndrome patients has been highest following surgery. Trauma is also a frequently reported associated event, although it is an extraordinarily weak causative factor. Among the sporadic cases, pregnant and postpartum women have occasionally developed desmoids [3].

Pathology

Desmoid tumors can arise from any body site and infiltrate neighboring tissues. In most cases, the tumor is confined to the musculature and the overlying aponeurosis or fascia. Occasional lesions may involve the periosteum and even lead to bone erosion, thereby confusing it with desmoplastic fibroma of the bone [15]. These tumors are distinct and separate from the broad spectrum of lesions categorized as variants of benign fibromatoses, such as Dupuytren's contracture, plantar fibromatosis, knuckle pads, keloids, and Peyronie's disease.

Macroscopically, most tumors measure 5 to 10 cm in greatest dimensions and have the appearance of a hard lump typically infiltrating and adhering to the local tissue. Examination of a transected specimen usually reveals a glistening, white, coarsely trabeculated surface resembling scar tissue, and the appearance of a capsule is often misleading because the tumor infiltration may extend well beyond the apparently circumscribed mass. It is often difficult to distinguish recurrent fibromatosis from scar tissue resulting from prior surgical excision.

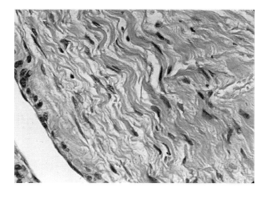

Fig. 1. Interlacing bundles of fibroblasts are shown in a case of extra-abdominal desmoid. Note that they are separated by varying amounts of collagen, with limited cell-to-cell contact (hematoxylin-eosin, original magnification × 100).

Desmoid tumors are composed of normal-appearing fibroblastic cells proliferating in an abundant fibrous stroma. Microscopically, the proliferation consists of elongated, slender, spindle-shaped cells of uniform appearance surrounded and separated from one another by abundant collagen, with little or no cell-to-cell contact (Fig. 1) [15]. The nuclei of the large fibroblasts show considerable pleomorphism, with notable mitotic activity and should not be mistaken for a fibrosarcoma. Unlike in fibrosarcomas, macrophages, multinucleated giant cells, and widespread lymphocytes are characteristic manifestations of desmoids. There is characteristically sparse cellularity, few mitoses, and rare necrosis. The periphery of the tumorous lesions often infiltrate the muscle tissue, and remnants of striated muscle fibers are frequently entrapped and undergo atrophy, which may occasionally be mistaken for malignant change.

Cytogenetics of desmoids

Although most desmoids appear normal on cytogenetic studies, trisomies for chromosomes 8 or 20 have been reported in approximately 20% of cases [16–18]. These are characteristically found in only about 10% to 30% of the desmoid tumor cells in any one patient and are most likely to be secondary mutations. Of interest, some reports suggest that desmoids associated with trisomy 8 are at increased risk of subsequent local recurrence [18,19]. Desmoid tumors from FAP may occasionally demonstrate a deletion of the long arm of chromosome 5 [20,21].

Gene array expression profiling studies have identified distinct clustering of desmoid tumors compared with other soft tissue tumors in a study that was able to identify very distinct clustering of gene expression profiles for desmoids, leiomyosarcomas, synovial sarcomas, liposarcomas, schwannomas, and gastrointestinal stromal tumors. Some of the tumors histologically classified as malignant fibrous histiocytoma (a diagnostic category about which there is some uncertainty) segregated together on a molecular basis, whereas others did not, demonstrating the potential diagnostic power of this tool in histologically challenging cases [22].

Differential diagnosis

Box 1 presents the common histologic differentials of desmoids with their characteristic findings [15].

Box 1. Common histologic differentials of desmoids with their characteristic findings

Fibrosarcoma

- Uniformly cellular and cells are arranged in a consistent sweeping growth pattern often described as a herringbone pattern
- Cells are often overlapping and separated by less collagen
- Nuclei are more hyperchromatic and atypical
- Nucleoli are more prominent
- Obvious high mitotic counts throughout the tumor
- Can metastasize; has a better-defined pseudocapsule on MRI

Reactive fibroblastic proliferations

- Injury is the likely etiology
- Cytologically, cells are indistinguishable from those in fibromatosis
- Frequent focal hemorrhage and hemosiderin deposition present
- More variable growth pattern

Desmoplastic fibroma of bone

- Predominates in metaphyseal or diaphyseal portions of long bones
- Radiographic studies are most helpful in distinguishing

Myxoma or nodular fasciatis

- Lesions are usually paucicellular with cells separated by abundant myxoid matrix
- Prominent uniform whorled pattern

Fibrosarcomatous transformation of fibromatosis

- Foci of increased cellularity
- Sarcomatous changes of atypia and hyperchromasia

From Weiss SW, Goldblum JR. Fibromatosis. In: Soft tissue tumors. Philadelphia: Mosby; 2001. p. 327–8; with permission.

Natural history

The clinical behavior of these tumors is unpredictable. Most lesions are likely to progress and may need treatment, but hematogenous or lymph node metastases have not been reported. Multicentric disease and recurrence (or reactivation) at sites other than the primary location have been reported [13]. Although mortality is rare in patients with extra-abdominal disease, it has been observed in some head and neck lesions [13]. Many lesions progress and some are refractory to multiple surgical procedures and adjuvant therapy. Of interest, spontaneous regression (approximately 15%) has been observed, as has regression after biopsy.

Although incapable of metastasizing, these tumors can rarely cause death when they invade or compress a vital structure, such as occurs in tumors in the root of the neck or within the abdomen [23]. In most published series, the 5-year survival rate is better than 90% [15]. The reported recurrence rate is variable and ranges from as low as 19% to as high as 77% [15]. In the Enzinger and Shiraki [24] series, with a minimum of 10 years of follow-up, 57% of tumors recurred. In one of the largest reported series of extra-abdominal desmoid tumors, Rock and colleagues [25] noted a recurrence rate of 68% after initial treatment.

Imaging studies

Desmoid lesions usually present as a soft tissue mass that interrupts the adjacent intermuscular and soft tissue planes. These lesions can sometimes encroach on the adjacent bone and cause pressure erosions or superficial defects of the cortex. Sometimes a periosteal reaction consisting of "frond-like" spicules of bone may be found extending deep into the tumor [26].

MRI scans are helpful in the diagnosis and assessment of tumor extent before surgery. It is important to note that desmoid tumors often extend microscopically well beyond their macroscopic margins. Desmoid tumors have a similar attenuation to muscle on CT; hence, CT examinations are of limited use.

On MRI, the lesions may be hypointense or hyperintense relative to surrounding muscle on T1- and T2-weighted sequences and heterogeneous changes are common [13]. Signal intensity variations correlate with the distribution of collagen and the cellularity of each lesion. Although MRI reflects the histology of the tumor lesion with low T2 signal changes seen in the collagenous lesions, imaging characteristics are nonspecific. MRI, however, is an

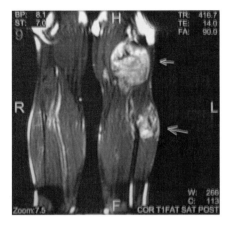

Fig. 2. A postcontrast, T1-weighted, fat-saturated, coronal MRI demonstrating multicentric desmoid tumors of the thigh that were proved with biopsy.

excellent means of outlining the extent of these lesions at presentation and for surveillance following the diagnosis and treatment. It is also helpful in assessing extent and relationship to neurovascular and other important functional structures before surgical resection [27–29].

Differentiating tumor progression from postsurgical fibrosis can be difficult during the early stages, and gadolinium contrast may help later because cellular areas will appear enhanced. Postoperative MRI at 3 months provides a baseline for comparison with later follow-up when recurrence may be suspected [13]. Of interest, multicentric and recurrent lesions are known to occur in the same anatomic region (Fig. 2); therefore, there seems to be a role for scanning the entire extremity after a diagnosis is made [30].

Clinical presentation

Extra-abdominal lesions are most common in patients between puberty and 40 years of age, with a peak incidence between the ages of 25 and 35 years [15]. Lesions are located in a variety of anatomic locations, with shoulder, chest wall, back, and thigh being the most frequent locations, in that order (Fig. 3).

Reitamo and colleagues [31] divided their series of 89 cases into four major age groups in which the sites of the tumor, the sex of the patient, or both were nonrandomly distributed (Box 2).

In most cases, lesions are firm and fixed to surrounding tissue. Most patients present with a poorly circumscribed mass that has grown insidiously.

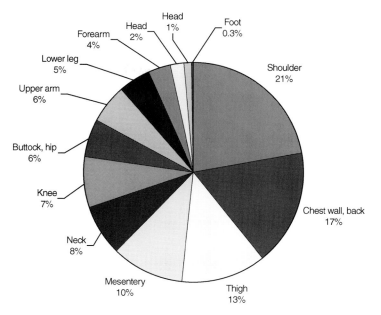

Fig. 3. A chart demonstrating the anatomic distribution of extra-abdominal desmoid tumors.

Moderate pain is a common complaint, and depending on the extent of invasion, there may be associated decreased mobility of adjacent joints. Neurologic manifestations including numbness, tingling, stabbing or shooting pain, or motor weakness may occur when the lesion has invaded or compressed local nerves. Other important factors that need to be addressed during general examination are outlined in Box 3.

Management

Management of desmoid tumors should be a multidisciplinary approach. Management should be aimed at achieving local control without the sacrifice of function or cosmesis. Surgery with a wide margin of resection remained the primary treatment modality until recent years and offered the best chance of avoiding recurrence; however, the indications and results of adjuvant therapies including chemotherapy and combination therapy (surgery with radiation or chemotherapy) are evolving. It is important to weigh the adversities of radical surgery and the various adjuvants against the potential morbidity of the tumor itself. It is very important, as with other musculoskeletal tumors, to have the patient evaluated in a multidisciplinary

---

Box 2. Four clinical groups describing patients who have desmoid lesions

Group I—Juvenile tumors: occurring predominantly in an extra-abdominal location with a distinct predilection for girls younger than 15 years of age

Group II—Fertile tumors: occurring exclusively as abdominal desmoid tumors in fertile females

Group III—Menopausal tumors: occurring predominantly in the abdomen, with an approximately equal number of men and women affected

Group IV—Senescent tumors: equally distributed between abdominal and extra-abdominal locations and equally frequent in both sexes

Data from Reitamo JJ, Hayry P, Nykyri E, et al. The desmoid tumor. I. Incidence, sex-, age- and anatomical distribution in the Finnish population. Am J Clin Pathol 1982; 77:665.

Box 3. Important features to be addressed during clinical examination of patients who have desmoids/fibromatosis

- Thorough family history for any relatives with similar lesions, and colonic carcinoma, polyps, or both should be noted
- Fundi should be examined for characteristic spots, and colonoscopy should be performed to rule out Gardner's syndrome in desmoid cases having positive family history and findings
- FAP/Gardner's syndrome patients who present with evidence of swellings are suspect for desmoids
- Intra-abdominal lesions may remain asymptomatic for long duration and may present with signs of intra-abdominal compression of viscera, requiring a thorough evaluation

fashion, including the orthopedic or surgical oncologist, radiation oncologist, and medical or pediatric oncologist.

Results of several recent studies are summarized in Table 1.

Surgery

When medically and technically feasible, surgery has been the traditional first-line therapy. Even when feasible, the morbidity and functional impairment resulting from surgery should be weighed against the expected behavior of the tumor and the potential efficacy of other treatments (Fig. 4). Multiple studies have documented excellent local control, with recurrence rates of 70% to 80% with wide negative margins [32,33]. Due to the tendency of these lesions to penetrate microscopically through adjacent tissues, however, wide margins are difficult to achieve without large soft tissue resections. Surgery is frequently combined with radiation because of the recurrence rate with surgery alone; however, a recent review of the surgical and radiation experience with desmoid tumors between 1983 and 1998 has questioned the need for radical surgery [34]. Twenty-two studies involving 780 patients with desmoid tumors were reviewed. The treatments evaluated included surgery, radiation, or a combination of both. Median follow-up of all studies combined was 6 years. Outcomes were superior in the arms including radiation therapy. Local control rates of surgery, surgery plus radiation, and radiation alone were 61%, 75%, and 78%, respectively.

Two potential prognostic factors are "margin status" and "disease status" (primary versus recur-

Table 1
Local control rates at 5 years

Investigators	N	Overall local control	Surgery: (n)	Surgery: local control	S + RT (n)	S + RT: local control	Radiation: (n)	Radiation: local control	Median follow-up (y)
Milan [32]	203	73%	163	72%	40	78%	—	—	11.25
Seoul [50]	24	88.5%	—	—	—	—	—	—	5.75
Heidelberg [51]	28	73%	—	—	26		2		3.8
U Florida [37]	65	83%	—	—	65	83%	—	—	6
Denmark [36]	72	73%	44	69%	28	78%	—	—	8
U Wash [38]	54	72%	19	53%	35	81%	—	—	3.25
MSKCC[a] (intra-abdominal)	24	73%	24	73%	—	—	—	—	5.17
MSKCC[a] [35] (extra-abdominal)	105	75%[a]	74	77%[a]	31	77%[a]	—	—	4.08
MGH [33]	107	74%	51	69%	41	72%	15	93%	5
MDACC [39]	75	78%	—	—	52	82%	23	69%	7.5
Germany [1]	345	—	—	—	262	79.6	83	81.4%	3.58

Abbreviations: MDACC, M.D. Anderson Cancer Center; MGH, Massachusetts General Hospital; MSKCC, Memorial Sloan-Kettering Cancer Center; S + RT, surgery and radiation; U, University of; —, no data.

[a] Data presented are local recurrence-free survival (all patients reported at 5 years), whereas surgery versus S + RT data factor all recurrences known by time of publications.

From Shih HA, Hornicek FJ, DeLaney TF. Fibromatosis: current strategies for treatment. Curr Opin Orthop 2003;14:405; with permission.

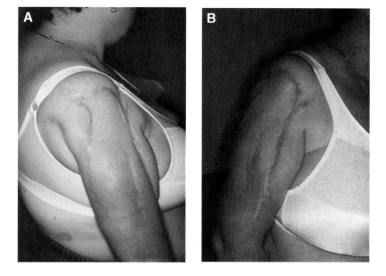

Fig. 4. (*A*, *B*) Clinical photographs of a patient who had recurrent desmoid tumors in the right arm and shoulder region. As evidenced by multiple scars, she underwent nine surgeries for recurrent lesions over an 11-year interval.

rent disease). The compiled results of Nuyttens and colleagues [34] showed improved local control rates with combined-modality therapy regardless of margin status. Among patients with negative margins, local control was 72% with surgery alone and 94% with surgery plus radiation ($P = 0.0048$). Likewise, patients with positive margins had local control rates of 41% with surgery alone and 75% with surgery plus radiation ($P < 0.0001$). Although primary tumors had better local control than recurrent tumors overall, subset analysis revealed that this was true only for positive-margin recurrent tumors treated by surgery alone. The addition of adjuvant radiation abrogated this difference. Recurrent tumors with negative margins had equivalent outcomes to their primary tumor counterparts following treatment by surgery or surgery plus radiation. The authors suggest that aggressive, highly morbid surgery cases should be replaced by more conservative resection and radiation therapy or radiation alone. Positive-margin surgery combined with radiation was no better than radiation alone.

Since the publication of the review by Nuyttens and colleagues [34] in 2000, few surgical series have been reported that would support primary surgery. Gronchi and coworkers [32] reported outcomes on 203 patients who had desmoid tumors who underwent gross total resection. Forty of these patients also received adjuvant radiation therapy. Median follow-up was more than 11 years. Disease-free survival was 73% and 70% at 5 and 10 years, respectively. Subset

analysis revealed improved outcomes among primary tumors compared with recurrent tumors ($P < 0.01$). At 5 and 10 years, disease-free survival was 81% and 76% in primary disease, and 59% and 59% in recurrent disease, respectively. There was a trend toward tumor recurrence only among recurrent tumors resected with a positive margin. No comment was made regarding the value of the radiation component except to say that there was no difference in outcome. Merchant and colleagues [35] from Memorial Sloan-Kettering Cancer Center reported a series of 105 patients who had primary desmoid tumors of extra-abdominal sites largely undergoing surgical management alone. With two exceptions, all patients underwent gross total resection, and local recurrence-free survival at 5 years was 75%. There was no difference in local recurrence between negative margins and microscopic residual disease, and no benefit was seen in the 31 patients who received adjuvant radiation compared with surgery alone. Sorensen and colleagues [36] reported the results of a study of 72 patients who had desmoid tumors treated by surgery alone. The disease was controlled in 73% of patients at 5 years. Multivariate analysis showed predictors for local recurrence included tumors larger than 4 cm, inadequate margin, age younger than 32 years, and extra-compartmental location. These reports support the case for definitive surgical management and make consideration for primary radiation a less-than-clear decision.

Radiation therapy

External beam radiation therapy has mainly been employed (1) in patients with unresectable disease, (2) to avoid mutilating surgery, (3) for gross residual tumor, and (4) for positive or equivocal margins following surgery. There are several recent studies that continue to support the efficacy of radiation therapy as primary or adjuvant therapy with surgery. Outcomes of 65 patients treated at the University of Florida in Gainesville with radiation or surgery plus radiation suggest that radiation alone can provide excellent local control and additional surgery does not add benefit in treatment of primary or recurrent tumors [37]. Regardless of therapy, primary tumors fared better than recurrent disease: local control rates at 5 years were 96% versus 75%, respectively. In a retrospective analysis of surgical outcomes with or without the addition of radiation, Jelinek and co-workers [38] reported a local control rate of 53% in 19 patients undergoing surgery alone compared with 81% in 35 patients receiving surgery and radiation (median dose, 57 Gy), supporting a clear role for adjuvant radiation.

Compilation of available data suggests an optimal radiation dose between 50 and 60 Gy. Doses of 17.5 to 35 Gy among 5 patients resulted in local failure in 3 patients. A total of 188 patients treated with radiation drawn from 10 articles resulted in 42 failures with no appreciable difference between 50 and 60 Gy compared with greater than 60 Gy [34,37, 39,40]. Significant increase in radiation morbidity is caused with doses greater than 60 Gy, especially in cases involving periosteal stripping, bone curettage, or where lymphatic drainage has been compromised. Possible complications of external beam radio-

therapy include growth arrest, fibrosis, edema, skin ulceration, cellulitis, pathologic fracture, secondary cancer, and neurologic changes including paresthesias and paresis.

Chemotherapy and other pharmacotherapy for desmoid tumors

Cytotoxic and noncytotoxic chemotherapeutic agents have been employed as adjuvants for the treatment of desmoids. Frequently, intra-abdominal and mesenteric tumors and large-extremity tumors are good candidates for medical therapy because of their poor candidacy for surgical or radiation management. An excellent review of the various drug approaches to desmoid tumors has recently been published [41].

Weiss and Lackman [42] employed vinblastine and methotrexate in eight patients who were not candidates for conservative surgery (Fig. 5). They reported symptomatic relief in all, with two complete remissions and four partial remissions. Low-dose combination chemotherapy has subsequently proved to have a 70% relapse-free interval at 10 years. A major advantage of low-dose chemotherapy is that it is the only treatment without permanent side effects. The medications are safe and cause no secondary malignancy. They are given in doses that cause minimal symptoms and do not normally cause marrow suppression. As such, chemotherapy in low doses is an excellent first round of treatment for any patient in whom contemplated local treatment has significant morbidity.

Clinical benefit is typically much higher than objective responses. Doxorubicin-based regimens

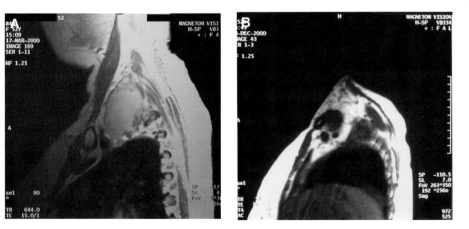

Fig. 5. MRI of a patient who had a recurrent desmoid tumor at the base of the neck. (*A*) The tumor before chemotherapy. (*B*) The tumor 9 months later, after chemotherapy, with an evident decrease in tumor size.

were initially designed based on their efficacy with sarcomas. These drug combinations have been partially successful; however, responses may be delayed and long-term therapy of at least 1 year is generally recommended. This treatment has now become less popular in view of the potential dangers of these drugs in the context of benign disease. In view of its good response rate and reduced toxicity, the current favored chemotherapy combination is methotrexate and vinblastine or its slightly less neurotoxic variation of methotrexate and vinorelbine. Other regimens include the use of doxorubicin, combination therapy with vincristine, dactinomycin, plus cyclophosphamide, and doxorubicin plus dacarbazine [43,44].

Concerns over the potential morbidity resulting from cytotoxic agents has led to an increasing interest in noncytotoxic agents including tamoxifen, testolactone, and the nonsteroidal anti-inflammatory drugs. Hormonal therapy, most commonly tamoxifen, has been used by most physicians. It is based on the rationale that desmoid tumors are more common and generally more aggressive in women compared with men and in premenopausal women compared with postmenopausal women [31]. Clinical response rates are approximately 50% and include a large proportion of recurrent tumors that had previously been treated with surgery or radiation [41]. It is unfortunate that long-term control of greater than 5 years has been low. Tamoxifen is favored in patients who have failed or who are poor candidates for the standard approaches. There are very limited data regarding the use of other hormonal agents such as progesterone, testolactone, and goserelin.

Nonsteroidal anti-inflammatory agents such as sulindac have been reported in largely anecdotal experiences to induce partial responses [41]. In a study by Tsukada and colleagues [45], 14 patients were treated with sulindac. Only 1 experienced a complete response, whereas 7 others experienced partial responses. The mechanism of action is hypothesized to be by way of cyclooxygenase inhibition, preventing activation of ornithine decarboxylase and causing decreases in cAMP and proliferative signals. Addition of cyclooxygenase-2 inhibitor in cell culture and in a mouse model for aggressive fibromatosis has shown decreases in cell proliferation and resultant smaller tumors [46]. Interferons, with or without retinoic acid, have been tried in a limited number of studies. In vitro findings of antiproliferative effect with this therapy make this treatment attractive, particularly in the adjuvant setting of high-risk disease [41].

Novel approaches

In their study of nine patients with treatment-refractory disease who had exhausted surgical, radiation, and other medical therapy options, Mace and coworkers [47] were able to demonstrate that all lesions expressed platelet-derived growth factor receptors. Two of the patients with recurrent disease underwent a trial with the tyrosine kinase inhibitor imatinib mesylate and experienced a partial response, with improved quality of life at 9 and 11 months.

Expression of somatostatin receptor subtype 2 has been demonstrated in some cases of desmoids; these patients have been treated with a yttrium 90–labeled somatostatin analog to cause disease stabilization and halt progression of disease [48]. Clark [49] successfully reported intralesional delivery (of ethanol and acetic acid or acetic acid alone) by CT guidance in two cases of bulky desmoid tumors, with significant regression of disease at last follow-up of 2 years.

Summary

Desmoids are a challenging group of lesions with variable biologic behavior and local morbidity but with no metastatic potential. Modern treatment involves a multidisciplinary and individualized approach based on the location, extent, and status of recurrence. Surgery continues to be a popular therapy for small resectable tumors. Radiation is also an effective alternative; however, its potential carcinogenic side effects must be weighed carefully in the context of young patients. Low-dose chemotherapy with methotrexate and vinblastine remains a noninvasive and safe treatment with a 10-year relapse-free rate of 70%. It is clear that desmoid tumors represent an extremely mixed population of tumors with very benign to very aggressive behavior. With better understanding of the molecular and genetic basis of this disease, it is hoped that more targeted therapies with minimal toxicity profiles will become available and become the preferred therapy.

References

[1] Micke O, Seegenschmiedt MH. Radiation therapy for aggressive fibromatosis (desmoid tumors): results of a national Patterns of Care Study. Int J Radiat Oncol Biol Phys 2005;61:882–91.

[2] MacFarlane J. Clinical reports of the surgical practice of the Glasgow Royal Infirmary. 1832. p. 63–7.

[3] Shih HA, Hornicek FJ, DeLaney TF. Fibromatosis: current strategies for treatment. Curr Opin Orthop 2003;14:405–12.

[4] Muller J. Ueber den feinern Bau und die Formen der krankhaften. Geschwulste 1838.

[5] Griffioen G, Bus PJ, Vasen HF, et al. Extracolonic manifestations of familial adenomatous polyposis: desmoid tumours, and upper gastrointestinal adenomas and carcinomas. Scand J Gastroenterol Suppl 1998; 225:85–91.

[6] Bertario L, Russo A, Sala P, et al. Multiple approach to the exploration of genotype-phenotype correlations in familial adenomatous polyposis. J Clin Oncol 2003; 21:1698–707.

[7] Clark SK, Phillips RK. Desmoids in familial adenomatous polyposis. Br J Surg 1996;83:1494–504.

[8] Hayry P, Reitamo JJ, Totterman S, et al. The desmoid tumor. II. Analysis of factors possibly contributing to the etiology and growth behavior. Am J Clin Pathol 1982;77:674–80.

[9] Alman BA, Goldberg MJ, Naber SP, et al. Aggressive fibromatosis. J Pediatr Orthop 1992;12:1–10.

[10] Kinzler KW, Nilbert MC, Vogelstein B, et al. Identification of a gene located at chromosome 5q21 that is mutated in colorectal cancers. Science 1991;251: 1366–70.

[11] Alman BA, Li C, Pajerski ME, et al. Increased beta-catenin protein and somatic APC mutations in sporadic aggressive fibromatoses (desmoid tumors). Am J Pathol 1997;151:329–34.

[12] Giarola M, Wells D, Mondini P, et al. Mutations of adenomatous polyposis coli (APC) gene are uncommon in sporadic desmoid tumours. Br J Cancer 1998; 78:582–7.

[13] Dormans JP, Spiegel D, Meyer J, et al. Fibromatoses in childhood: the desmoid/fibromatosis complex. Med Pediatr Oncol 2001;37:126–31.

[14] Kong Y, Poon R, Nadesan P, et al. Matrix metalloproteinase activity modulates tumor size, cell motility, and cell invasiveness in murine aggressive fibromatosis. Cancer Res 2004;64:5795–803.

[15] Weiss SW, Goldblum JR. Fibromatosis. In: Enzinger FM, Weiss SW, editors. Soft tissue tumors. Philadelphia: Mosby; 2001. p. 309–46.

[16] Dal Cin P, Sciot R, Aly MS, et al. Some desmoid tumors are characterized by trisomy 8. Genes Chromosomes Cancer 1994;10:131–5.

[17] Mertens F, Willen H, Rydholm A, et al. Trisomy 20 is a primary chromosome aberration in desmoid tumors. Int J Cancer 1995;63:527–9.

[18] Fletcher JA, Naeem R, Xiao S, et al. Chromosome aberrations in desmoid tumors. Trisomy 8 may be a predictor of recurrence. Cancer Genet Cytogenet 1995; 79:139–43.

[19] Kouho H, Aoki T, Hisaoka M, et al. Clinicopathological and interphase cytogenetic analysis of desmoid tumours. Histopathology 1997;31:336–41.

[20] Bridge JA, Sreekantaiah C, Mouron B, et al. Clonal chromosomal abnormalities in desmoid tumors.

[21] Dangel A, Meloni AM, Lynch HT, et al. Deletion (5q) in a desmoid tumor of a patient with Gardner's syndrome. Cancer Genet Cytogenet 1994;78:94–8.

[22] Skubitz KM, Skubitz AP. Characterization of sarcomas by means of gene expression. J Lab Clin Med 2004;144:78–91.

[23] Allen PW. The fibromatoses: a clinicopathologic classification based on 140 cases. Am J Surg Pathol 1977;1:255–70.

[24] Enzinger FM, Shiraki M. Musculo-aponeurotic fibromatosis of the shoulder girdle (extra-abdominal desmoid). Analysis of thirty cases followed up for ten or more years. Cancer 1967;20:1131–40.

[25] Rock MG, Pritchard DJ, Reiman HM, et al. Extraabdominal desmoid tumors. J Bone Joint Surg Am 1984;66:1369–74.

[26] Abramowitz D, Zornoza J, Ayala AG, et al. Soft-tissue desmoid tumors: radiographic bone changes. Radiology 1983;146:11–3.

[27] Tanaka H, Harasawa A, Furui S. Usefulness of MR imaging in assessment of tumor extent of aggressive fibromatosis. Radiat Med 2005;23:111–5.

[28] Liu P, Thorner P. MRI of fibromatosis: with pathologic correlation. Pediatr Radiol 1992;22:587–9.

[29] Vandevenne JE, De Schepper AM, De Beuckeleer L, et al. New concepts in understanding evolution of desmoid tumors: MR imaging of 30 lesions. Eur Radiol 1997;7:1013–9.

[30] Sundaram M, Duffrin H, McGuire MH, et al. Synchronous multicentric desmoid tumors (aggressive fibromatosis) of the extremities. Skeletal Radiol 1988;17: 16–9.

[31] Reitamo JJ, Hayry P, Nykyri E, et al. The desmoid tumor. I. Incidence, sex-, age- and anatomical distribution in the Finnish population. Am J Clin Pathol 1982;77:665–73.

[32] Gronchi A, Casali PG, Mariani L, et al. Quality of surgery and outcome in extra-abdominal aggressive fibromatosis: a series of patients surgically treated at a single institution. J Clin Oncol 2003;21: 1390–7.

[33] Spear MA, Jennings LC, Mankin HJ, et al. Individualizing management of aggressive fibromatoses. Int J Radiat Oncol Biol Phys 1998;40:637–45.

[34] Nuyttens JJ, Rust PF, Thomas Jr CR, et al. Surgery versus radiation therapy for patients with aggressive fibromatosis or desmoid tumors: a comparative review of 22 articles. Cancer 2000;88:1517–23.

[35] Merchant NB, Lewis JJ, Woodruff JM, et al. Extremity and trunk desmoid tumors: a multifactorial analysis of outcome. Cancer 1999;86:2045–52.

[36] Sorensen A, Keller J, Nielsen OS, et al. Treatment of aggressive fibromatosis: a retrospective study of 72 patients followed for 1–27 years. Acta Orthop Scand 2002;73:213–9.

[37] Zlotecki RA, Scarborough MT, Morris CG, et al. External beam radiotherapy for primary and adjuvant

Implications for histopathogenesis. Cancer 1992;69: 430–6.

management of aggressive fibromatosis. Int J Radiat Oncol Biol Phys 2002;54:177–81.

[38] Jelinek JA, Stelzer KJ, Conrad E, et al. The efficacy of radiotherapy as postoperative treatment for desmoid tumors. Int J Radiat Oncol Biol Phys 2001;50:121–5.

[39] Ballo MT, Zagars GK, Pollack A. Radiation therapy in the management of desmoid tumors. Int J Radiat Oncol Biol Phys 1998;42:1007–14.

[40] Acker JC, Bossen EH, Halperin EC. The management of desmoid tumors. Int J Radiat Oncol Biol Phys 1993;26:851–8.

[41] Janinis J, Patriki M, Vini L, et al. The pharmacological treatment of aggressive fibromatosis: a systematic review. Ann Oncol 2003;14:181–90.

[42] Weiss AJ, Lackman RD. Low-dose chemotherapy of desmoid tumors. Cancer 1989;64:1192–4.

[43] Stein R. Chemotherapeutic response in fibromatosis of the neck. J Pediatr 1977;90:482–3.

[44] Seiter K, Kemeny N. Successful treatment of a desmoid tumor with doxorubicin. Cancer 1993;71:2242–4.

[45] Tsukada K, Church JM, Jagelman DG, et al. Non- cytotoxic drug therapy for intra-abdominal desmoid tumor in patients with familial adenomatous polyposis. Dis Colon Rectum 1992;35:29–33.

[46] Poon R, Smits R, Li C, et al. Cyclooxygenase-two (COX-2) modulates proliferation in aggressive fibromatosis (desmoid tumor). Oncogene 2001;20:451–60.

[47] Mace J, Sybil Biermann J, Sondak V, et al. Response of extraabdominal desmoid tumors to therapy with imatinib mesylate. Cancer 2002;95:2373–9.

[48] De Pas T, Bodei L, Pelosi G, et al. Peptide receptor radiotherapy: a new option for the management of aggressive fibromatosis on behalf of the Italian Sarcoma Group. Br J Cancer 2003;88:645–7.

[49] Clark TW. Percutaneous chemical ablation of desmoid tumors. J Vasc Interv Radiol 2003;14:629–34.

[50] Park H, Pyo HR, Shin KH, et al. Radiation treatment for aggressive fibromatosis: findings from observed patterns of local failure. Oncology 2003;64:346–52.

[51] Schulz-Ertner D, Zierhut D, Mende U, et al. The role of radiation therapy in the management of desmoid tumors. Strahlenther Onkol 2002;178:78–83.

ORTHOPEDIC
CLINICS
OF NORTH AMERICA

Orthop Clin N Am 37 (2006) 65 – 74

Massive Allograft Use in Orthopedic Oncology

D. Luis Muscolo, MD*, Miguel A. Ayerza, MD, Luis A. Aponte-Tinao, MD

Institute of Orthopedics "Carlos E. Ottolenghi," Italian Hospital of Buenos Aires, Potosí 4215 (1199), Buenos Aires, Argentina

Tumor excision with wide surgical margins is the primary treatment of aggressive or recurrent benign bone tumors and malignant bone sarcomas. This treatment requires a surgical resection that has a potential large residual osseous defect. As diagnostic and therapeutic techniques improve, patients who have musculoskeletal sarcomas can expect increased survivals, decreased complications and side effects, and an improved quality of life. Functional longevity of the reconstruction, however, becomes a major concern, especially in young and physically active patients.

Due to concerns involving the durability of prosthetic materials and the increasing survivorship of patients who have sarcomas, emphasis has been placed on biologic reconstructive alternatives. Allograft transplantation is a functional reconstructive option for large-extremity osseous defects. Advantages of allografts [1–7] include the possibility of supporting mechanical loads and attaching host ligaments and muscles to the allografts. In addition, grafts are readily available from tissue banks and can be matched to the size of the resected bone. Another potential advantage of allografts over synthetic materials is that they may be progressively incorporated by the host. Disadvantages of using bone allografts include possible disease transmission, host–donor junction complications, and negative effects on the strength and elastic modulus of the graft due to processing techniques.

Osteoarticular allografts

Total condylar allografts

Total condylar osteoarticular allografts are used for reconstruction of one side of the joint after tumor resection, prohibiting the need for sacrificing the other side of the joint not compromised by the tumor (Figs. 1 and 2). Osteoarticular grafts are also possible in replacing articular surfaces for which prostheses are not readily available such as the distal tibia (Fig. 3) or distal radius. The availability of soft tissues on the allografts is an advantage for attaching the host tendons or ligaments.

Although osteoarticular allografts are ideal material for biologic reconstruction of skeletal defects, biomechanically and biologically related complications including bone graft fractures and resorption, cartilage degeneration, joint instability, and delayed bone union or nonunion still occur. These biomechanically related complications can be grouped into two main categories: (1) geometric matching between the allograft and the host defect and (2) stability achieved during surgery of the allograft–host bone and soft tissue junction sites. Anatomic and dimensional matching of the articular surface, adequate joint stability obtained by host–donor soft tissue repair, and joint alignment have been associated with minor degenerative changes at the articular surface [5,6,8,9]. Clinicopathologic studies performed in human-retrieved allografts found earlier and more advanced degenerative changes in articular cartilage in specimens retrieved from patients who had an unstable joint compared with those who had a stable joint [8].

Poor anatomic matching of size and shape between the host defect and the graft can significantly

* Corresponding author.

E-mail address: luis.muscolo@hospitalitaliano.org.ar
(D.L. Muscolo).

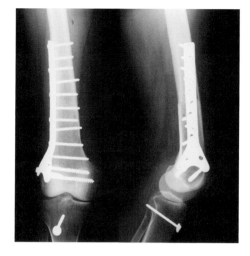

Fig. 1. Anteroposterior (*left*) and lateral (*right*) radiographs of a distal femur osteoarticular allograft made 5 years after implantation that show a well-healed allograft–host junction.

alter joint kinematics and load distribution, leading to bone resorption or joint degeneration. To improve accuracy in size matching between the donor and host, the authors developed measurable parameters based on CT scans of the distal femur and the proximal tibia. In the axial view of the distal femur, the authors measure the maximum total width and anteroposterior width of the medial and lateral

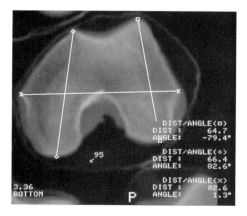

Fig. 3. Preoperative (*left*) and postoperative (*right*) anteroposterior radiographs of a patient who had a Ewing's sarcoma of the distal tibia in which an osteoarticular allograft was performed that show a good osteotomy healing and minor deterioration of the joint.

condyles (Fig. 4) and the width of the intercondylar notch (Fig. 5). In the proximal tibia, the maximum total width and the anteroposterior width of the medial and lateral plateaus are measured (Fig. 6). These measurements are available in the authors' hospital-based bone bank and allow optimal selection

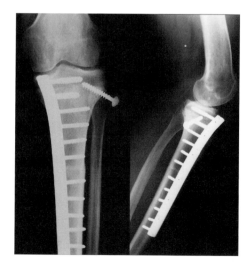

Fig. 2. Anteroposterior (*left*) and lateral (*right*) radiograph controls made 6 years after implantation of a proximal tibia osteoarticular allograft that show an adequate articular space and solid union of the osteotomy.

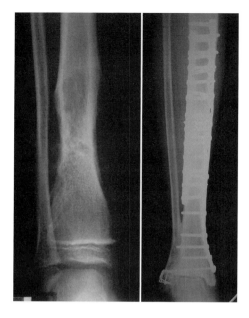

Fig. 4. Axial view of a distal femur allograft CT scan before implantation that shows the measure of the maximum total width and the anteroposterior width of the medial and lateral condyles.

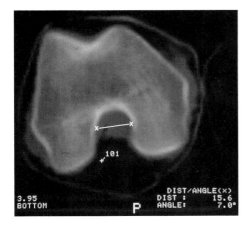

Fig. 5. Axial view of a distal femur allograft CT scan before implantation that shows the measure of the width of the intercondylar notch.

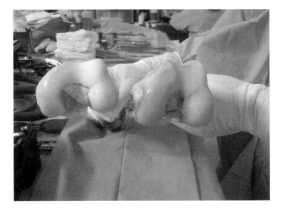

Fig. 7. Intraoperative photograph that shows two distal femur allografts with similar width but different anteroposterior width of the medial and lateral condyles and of the intercondylar notch.

of the graft to match the patient (Fig. 7). Selection and placement of a graft not anatomically matching the size of the osteoarticular defect may alter joint kinematics and pressure distribution, which in turn may reduce the functional life of the graft.

Although the allograft–host union depends on a variety of biologic factors involving immunology, tissue typing, or graft preservation, a successful union also relies on the availability to overcome biomechanical problems. In allograft reconstruction, there is high stress at the osteotomy site between the host and allograft bone. If the graft is not protected with appropriate internal fixation, then nonunion or fracture may result. Under these circumstances, if the graft is protected and a solid union is achieved, then it may be able to support continuous mechanical

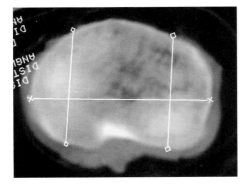

Fig. 6. Axial view of a proximal tibia allograft CT scan before implantation showing how the authors measure the maximum total width and the anteroposterior width of the medial and lateral plateaus.

loads. Chemotherapy is always a major concern when an allograft reconstruction is considered. The antiblastic toxicity of chemotherapeutic drugs is known to have an inhibitory effect on allograft union and repair in animals [10]. Studies performed in human-retrieved allografts seem to associate preoperative chemotherapy with retarded host–donor union [8]. In a recent report of 200 osteoarticular allografts that were analyzed (64 without chemotherapy and 126 with chemotherapy), the nonunion rate was markedly increased in patients who received chemotherapy (32% versus 12%), with no differences in infection or fracture rate [11]. Excessive motion at the host–graft interface as a result of an inadequate fixation can inhibit bone union. Further, the biologic incorporation of a cortical allograft is a slow process of induction requiring creeping substitution. A stable host–graft interface with a high degree of contact and a rigid surgical construct may be particularly important to obtain long-term survival of an allograft [5,7,9] because the deleterious effect of chemotherapy seems to be a reversible process [10] and allograft healing may occur at the end of the chemotherapy period.

Reconstruction of the ligaments, tendons, and joint capsule must be meticulous and precise because the longevity of these grafts is related, in part, to the stability of the joint. Care must be taken to avoid malalignment that will put greater stress on the allograft cartilage.

The allografts are selected based on age, sex, height, and CT scans of the patient and are compared with data available on the donor to achieve the best anatomic match. The grafts are taken out of their packaging and placed directly in a warm solution. After being thawed, the donor bone is cut to the proper length and soft tissue structures such as cruciate ligaments, collateral ligaments, and posterior capsule are prepared for implantation. Through an extended anterior-medial approach of the knee, the extensor mechanism is released and the bone tumor is resected with an adequate margin of normal tissue according to preoperative staging studies. All resections are intra-articular and intracompartmental. At the time of allograft implantation, a rigid fixation of the host–donor junction is obtained. A transverse osteotomy is used in every case. Originally, in the 1970s and early 1980s, this junction site was autografted with cortical cancellous bone graft to increase healing. At this time, osteoarticular allografts were performed mainly for aggressive benign tumors (giant cell tumor). When this type of reconstruction was in malignant bone tumors, no autograft was used to decrease morbidity. The authors observed that when rigid fixation was achieved even though autograft was not used, complete healing of the osteotomy was obtained. This finding led the authors to discontinue their use of autograft. Uniform cortical contact, compression of the osteotomy gap, and rotational stability were noted to be better when internal fixation plates and screws were used. A second anterior plate is often necessary to provide rigid fixation when long allografts are used. With the intention to obtain a solid allograft construct, the internal fixation should span the entire length of the allograft in all cases. Soft tissues from the allograft are attached to corresponding host tissues for improved stability. These soft tissue reconstructions include the repair of the posterior capsule, anterior and posterior cruciate ligaments, medial and lateral collateral ligaments, and patellar ligament in tibial allografts. Reattachment of the allograft tissue to the corresponding host tissue is performed through a direct lateral-lateral continuous suture. Both host's menisci are preserved and reattached to the osteoarticular allograft tissue.

In a review of 386 patients treated with an osteoarticular allograft, Mankin and colleagues [4] reported excellent or good results (according to their grading system) for 73% of the patients when followed for more than 2 years. Muscolo and coworkers [9], in a study of 114 patients treated with an osteoarticular allograft of the distal femur or the proximal tibia, reported that the 5-year survival rate for the grafts was 73% and the rate of limb preservation was 93%, with a mean radiographic score of 83%. One third of the patients had radiographic evidence of articular deterioration after 5 years. Mnaymneh and

colleagues [12] reviewed the cases of 83 patients treated with a distal femoral osteoarticular allograft and followed for a minimum of 2 years. According to the grading system of Mankin and colleagues [4], the results were good or excellent for 70% of the 53 patients treated without chemotherapy compared with only 53% of the 30 patients treated with chemotherapy. In a recent report [13], 80 osteoarticular distal femur allograft (see Fig. 5) reconstructions were followed for a mean of 82 months. Overall allograft survival was 78% at 5 and 10 years, and the rate of allograft survival without the need for subsequent knee prosthesis resurfacing was 71% at 5 and 10 years. Age, sex, the use of chemotherapy, or the percentage of resected femur did not have a statistically significant effect on the overall allograft survival rates. Those patients who retained the original allograft had excellent functional and radiographic results.

Unlike the prosthesis, osteoarticular proximal tibia allograft provides an anatomic and biologic reconstruction of the extensor mechanism of the knee. Clohisy and Mankin [14] reported on 16 patients who received a proximal tibia allograft with an average of 90° of active motion of the knee, having a Musculoskeletal Tumor Society (MSTS) score of good or excellent in 9 patients. Five patients had extension strength in the involved knee equivalent to that in the contralateral knee, 6 had strength that was greater than antigravity but less than normal, and 3 had only antigravity strength. Brien and colleagues [15] evaluated 17 proximal tibia reconstructions. Although 10 patients had excellent or good results, they noted that the most common problem was mild instability and extensor weakness. A recent study [16] reviewed 38 patients treated with a proximal tibial osteoarticular allograft. Results were satisfactory (good or excellent) in 66% of the patients, with no significant difference between patients who received chemotherapy and those who did not.

Osteoarticular allografts in the upper limb are used less frequently than other types of osteoarticular allografts. Gebhardt and colleagues [17] reported that 12 of 20 patients (60%) treated with proximal humeral allografts had a satisfactory result. Getty and Peabody [18], in a study of 16 patients, reported that the Kaplan-Meier survival curve demonstrated a 68% 5-year rate of survival of the allografts; however, the functional limitations and an extremely high rate of complications led those investigators to abandon the routine use of osteoarticular allografts to replace the proximal aspect of the humerus. In a recent report [19] of 31 patients, however, 23 of the allograft canals filled with cement showed a survival of 78% at 5 years. These investigators concluded that this technique is a reliable reconstructive option for proximal humerus reconstruction.

Osteoarticular allografts of the distal part of the radius replace an articular surface for which prostheses are not readily available. Kocher and colleagues [20] reported on 24 patients who had reconstruction of the distal aspect of the radius with an osteoarticular allograft, done mostly after resection of a giant cell tumor. Eight eventually needed a revision, most frequently because of a fracture (4 patients) or wrist pain (2 patients). There were 14 other complications necessitating additional operative management. Of the 16 patients in whom the graft survived, 3 had no functional limitation, 9 reported limitation only with strenuous activities, and 4 had limitations in the ability to perform moderate activities.

Hemicondylar allografts

Hemicondylar osteoarticular allografts are mainly used following resection of a benign aggressive tumor (such as giant cell tumor) around the knee (Figs. 8 and 9) or a malignant tumor (such as an osteosarcoma) with limited compromise to one condyle and with clearly defined tumor margins. The surgical technique is demanding. As the authors described in the section on total condylar allografts, selection of the closest anatomic match between the host and donor is crucial. In addition, even if an ideal hemicondylar graft is selected, improper surgical

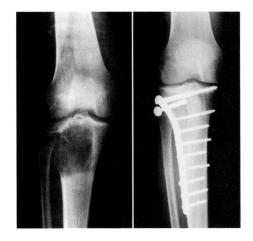

Fig. 9. Anteroposterior radiograph of a patient who had a giant cell tumor of the external tibial plateau before (*left*) and after (*right*) reconstruction with a unicompartmental tibial allograft fixed with a buttress plate. Note the healing of the osteotomy and the alignment 5 years after reconstruction.

placement could adversely affect the entire effort of the graft size and shape matching scheme. Distal or proximal malposition offset would lead to inappropriate loading of the articular surface, with a consequent varus or valgus deformity of the joint.

The stability provided by the soft tissue reconstruction is also an important factor for joint stability after graft placement, especially if the graft size is not properly matched. The ligament stability after the allograft replacement is changed by tightening or releasing it, but this type of reconstruction is more demanding because one side of the ligament is normal.

In a recent report [21] of 40 unicompartmental osteoarticular allografts of the knee followed for a mean of 10 years, the survival rate at 5 years was 85%. There were six failures: two local recurrences, two infections, one fracture, and one massive resorption. Unicompartmental allografts appear to be an alternative in situations in which the reconstruction is limited to one compartment.

Intercalary allografts

Allograft arthrodesis

Arthrodesis is at present reserved for reconstruction after extra-articular resection or for salvage procedures after failed reconstruction. The success of

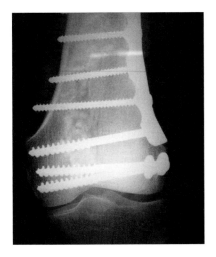

Fig. 8. Anteroposterior radiograph of a hemicondylar allograft of the distal femur after resection of a giant cell tumor.

allograft arthrodesis is not as good as intercalary segmental reconstruction.

Weiner and colleagues [22] reported that in 32 of 39 patients who had an allograft arthrodesis after resection of a tumor around the knee, the proximal and the distal allograft–host junction healed and the functional result was satisfactory. Mankin and colleagues [4], however, reported that after reviewing 71 patients who had an allograft arthrodesis, only 3% had an excellent result and 51% had a good result according to their scoring system. In a recent report [23] of a two-center study, 92 patients who had knee arthrodesis were analyzed. The results showed that complications were greater (infection, 20%; fracture, 25%; nonunion, 44%) and the outcome less successful than other types of reconstructions, suggesting that other approaches should be considered for this procedure. This high rate of complications could be explained, in part, by the loss of adjacent soft tissue from the wide resection, which may make healing more difficult and infection after reoperation more likely. In addition, the allografts implanted in replacement of the knee may not be strong enough to resist high rotational forces ordinarily acting on the knee. With adequate fixation and attention to detail, however, this procedure may still be indicated for patients who require an extra-articular resection.

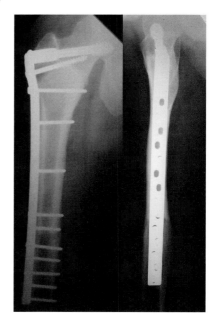

Fig. 11. Anteroposterior (*left*) and lateral (*right*) radiographs 4 years after resection of an osteosarcoma and reconstruction with a femur intercalary allograft shwoing both osteotomies healed with mature callus.

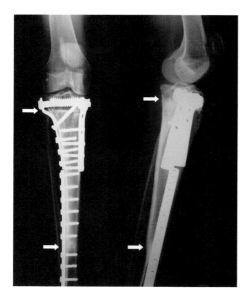

Fig. 10. Anteroposterior (*left*) and lateral (*right*) radiographs 15 years after transepiphyseal resection of an osteosarcoma located at the proximal tibia and reconstruction with an intercalary allograft that show healing of both host-to-graft junctions (*arrows*).

Intercalary segmental allografts

As imaging techniques improve, many tumors contained within the metadiaphyseal region of long bones may be treated by wide resection but with epiphyseal preservation [24–30]. Intercalary segmental allografts can be fixed to small epiphyseal host fragments, obtaining immediate limb stability and allowing active adjacent joint motion (Fig. 10). This methodology avoids complications associated with osteoarticular allografts, such as cartilage degeneration, joint collapse, or instability [8]. After healing of host–donor junctions, the graft may be incorporated progressively by the host (Fig. 11). This reconstruction can also be combined with a vascularized fibular graft to accelerate osseous union at the osteotomy sites [27].

The surgical procedure begins with resection of the lesion, including biopsy scars and with appropriate bone and soft tissue margins. The deep-frozen allograft segment is thawed, sized, and inserted to fit the bone defect. All allograft–host junctions are prepared with a transverse osteotomy. The authors prefer plates and screws over intramedullary nails for fixation of the grafts to achieve more rigid fixation. In cases where the thin epiphyseal segment is saved,

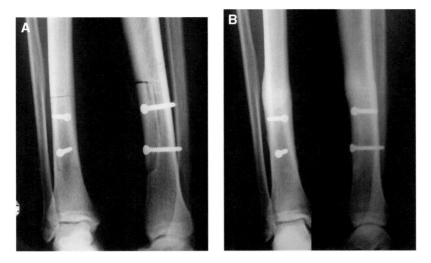

Fig. 12. A 35-year-old man with a parosteal osteosarcoma of the distal tibia in whom a hemicylindric allograft was performed after resection of a low-grade malignant bone tumor. (*A*) Anteroposterior (*left*) and lateral (*right*) radiographs of the patient immediately after surgery. (*B*) Anteroposterior (*left*) and lateral (*right*) radiographs 3 years after surgery showing graft incorporation without resorption.

only cancellous screws are used for fixation at the host–donor junction.

Ortiz-Cruz and colleagues [31] reported that 87 of 104 patients (84%) who were followed for at least 2 years had a successful result, with a 92% rate of limb salvage. They did not find any differences in nonunion between diaphyseal or metaphyseal bone or with different internal fixation. Cara and colleagues [32] reported a lower rate of satisfactory functional outcomes, with an excellent or good result in only 14 of 23 patients (61%). They reported nonunion only in the diaphyseal osteotomies. In a recent report [33] that reviewed 59 patients followed for a mean of 5 years, the 5-year survival rate was 79%, with no differences in allograft survival in patients receiving or not receiving adjuvant chemotherapy. The nonunion rate for diaphyseal junctions was higher (15%) than the rate for metaphyseal junctions (2%). Although some patients required reoperation because of allograft complications, it seems that the use of intercalary allograft clearly has a place in the reconstruction of a segmental defect created by the resection of a tumor in the diaphyseal or metaphyseal portion of the femur or tibia.

Hemicylindric intercalary allografts

Hemicylindric intercalary allografts may be used after resection of low-grade surface tumors (Fig. 12)

or to reconstruct the cortical window after intralesional curettage of a benign lesion (Fig. 13).

Deijkers and colleagues [34] reported on a series of 22 patients in whom a hemicortical allograft was performed after resection of a low-grade malignant bone tumor. There was no evidence of local recurrence, and all allografts incorporated completely with

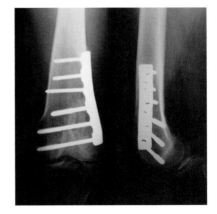

Fig. 13. Anteroposterior (*left*) and lateral (*right*) radiographs after intralesional curettage of a giant cell tumor of the distal femur. Treatment combined fragmented bone allograft to fill the cavity and a structural cortical allograft to reconstruct the cortical window, thus maintaining the articular surface of the host.

no fractures or infections. Ayerza and coworkers [35] reported a technique for reconstruction after intralesional curettage of giant cell tumor of the distal femur, combining fragmented bone allograft to fill the cavity and a structural cortical allograft to reconstruct the cortical window. This additional strut allograft buttresses the affected bone segment, restores the physiologic load, and avoids potential fractures due to abnormal cortical load transmission in patients treated with fragmented allograft alone. It also allows immediate partial weight bearing and contains the allografts chips within the bone.

Allograft–prosthesis composites

The resection and subsequent reconstruction using the combination of an allograft and a prosthesis (composite biologic implant) has become increasingly popular [1–5,7,36–38]. The advantages of allograft–prosthesis composites are that the bone stock is replaced and secure attachments for tendon insertions are provided without the need to rely on allograft articular cartilage, and the allograft does not need to be perfectly size matched to the host bone. Allografts provide tendinous attachments for reconstructions of the extensor mechanism in the knee, the rotator cuff in the shoulder, or the abductor muscles in the hip. Attachments of these muscular groups function better when repaired to allograft tendons than when they are attached to an endoprosthetic device.

At the authors' institution, the allograft is cut to the proper length on a separate, clean table at the same time that tumor resection is performed. The canal is prepared with the appropriate reamers. After the conventional prosthesis is cemented to the allograft, the composite is fixed to the host bone with plate and screws. The plate should expand the entire length of the allograft to minimize the risk of fracture (Fig. 14). Although some investigators report the use of a long stem extending beyond the length of the allograft to minimize the risk of fracture, the authors believe that this carries a significant part of the load to the distal part of the prosthesis, bypassing the allograft, henceforth delaying healing of the osteotomy and potentially leading to the resorption of the allograft. The final step of the reconstruction consists of reattachment of the host tendons to the allografts. When the authors analyzed their series of proximal femur composites, they found that most of the patients in whom the greater trochanter was reattached had a nonunion, whereas those patients who had a tendon-to-tendon repair had optimal

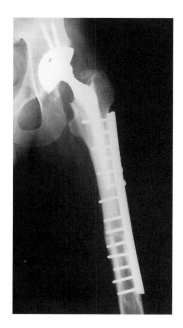

Fig. 14. Anteroposterior radiograph of a patient 6 years after resection of a Ewing's sarcoma of the proximal femur in whom an allograft–prosthetic composite was performed. Note that the plate expanded the entire length of the allograft to decrease the risk of fracture.

strength of the abductor mechanism without disruption. Tendon-to-tendon repair is recommended because it provides adequate healing.

Mankin and colleagues [4] reported 77% good or excellent results in 98 patients who had allograft–prosthesis composites followed for at least 2 years. Zehr and coworkers [37] found no significant differences in clinical function or longevity of the reconstructions when they compared 18 megaprostheses with 18 composites following resection of the proximal part of the femur. The 10-year survival rate was 58% in the megaprosthesis group and 76% in the composite group. The most common complication in the group treated with the megaprosthesis was instability, which occurred in 5 patients (28%). The main complication in the composite group was infection (3 patients). Langlais and colleagues [38] reported a survival rate of 81% at 10 years for composite prostheses compared with a rate of only 65% for megaprostheses. None of the composites had infection or dislocation.

Finally, in patients who have severe bone loss due to a failed endoprostheses who require revision, an allograft–prosthetic composite serves as an excellent

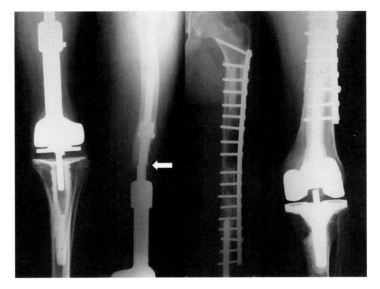

Fig. 15. Anteroposterior radiographs (*right*) of a patient in whom an allograft–prosthetic composite of the distal femur was performed because of a failed distal femur custom-expandable prosthesis (*left*) due to fracture of the femoral component (*arrow*). Note that 5 years after reconstruction, the osteotomy line is not visible (*right*).

long-term replacement without significant loss of function (Fig. 15) [39].

Summary

Allografts continue to be a very valuable alternative in orthopedic oncology. Improvements in anatomic matching, infection prevention, allograft fixation, soft tissue reconstructions, and rehabilitation protocols have greatly influenced predictability and longevity of massive allografts. These demanding reconstructions require time, an experienced group of orthopedic surgeons working at an institution with access to a large volume of patients, and a reliable, modern bone bank to select the appropriate graft for each individual under safe conditions. The benefit is to obtain a biologic reconstruction oriented to the present demand in orthopedic oncology: a reconstruction durable for many decades in patients cured of their disease.

References

[1] Gebhardt MC, Flugstad DI, Springfield DS, et al. The use of bone allografts for limb salvage in high-grade extremity osteosarcoma. Clin Orthop 1991;270: 181–96.

[2] Gitelis S, Heligman D, Quill G, et al. The use of large allografts for tumor reconstruction and salvage of the failed total hip arthroplasty. Clin Orthop 1988; 231:62–70.

[3] Mankin HJ, Gebhardt MC, Tomford WW. The use of frozen cadaveric allografts in the management of patients with bone tumors of the extremities. Orthop Clin N Am 1987;18:275–89.

[4] Mankin HJ, Gebhardt MC, Jennings LC, et al. Long-term results of allograft replacement in the management of bone tumors. Clin Orthop 1996;324:86–97.

[5] Muscolo DL, Petracchi LJ, Ayerza MA, et al. Massive femoral allografts followed for 22 to 36 years. J Bone Joint Surg Br 1992;74:887–92.

[6] Muscolo DL, Ayerza MA, Calabrese ME, et al. The use of a bone allograft for reconstruction after resection of giant-cell tumor close to the knee. J Bone Joint Surg Am 1993;75:1656–62.

[7] Ottolenghi CE, Muscolo DL, Maenza R. Bone defect reconstruction by massive allograft: technique and results of 51 cases followed for 5 to 32 years. In: Straub LR, Wilson PD, editors. Clinical trends in orthopaedics. New York: Thieme-Stratton; 1982. p. 171–83.

[8] Enneking WF, Campanacci DA. Retrieved human allografts. A clinicopathological study. J Bone Joint Surg Am 2001;83:971–86.

[9] Muscolo DL, Ayerza MA, Aponte-Tinao LA. Survivorship and radiographic analysis of knee osteoarticular allografts. Clin Orthop 2000;373:73–9.

[10] Friedlander GE, Tross RB, Doganis AC, et al. Effects of chemotherapeutic agents on bone. Short-term

methotrexate and doxorubicin (Adriamycin) treatment in a rat model. J Bone Joint Surg Am 1984;66:602 – 7.

[11] Hazan EJ, Hornicek FJ, Tomford WW, et al. The effect of adjuvant chemotherapy on osteoarticular allografts. Clin Orthop 2001;385:176 – 81.

[12] Mnaymneh W, Malinin TI, Lackman RD, et al. Massive distal femoral osteoarticular allografts after resection of bone tumors. Clin Orthop 1994;303: 103 – 15.

[13] Muscolo DL, Ayerza MA, Aponte-Tinao LA. The use of distal femoral osteoarticular allografts in limb salvage surgery. J Bone Joint Surg Am 2005, in press.

[14] Clohisy DR, Mankin HJ. Osteoarticular allografts for reconstruction after resection of a musculoskeletal tumor in the proximal end of the tibia. J Bone Joint Surg Am 1994;76:549 – 54.

[15] Brien EW, Terek RM, Healey JH, et al. Allograft reconstruction after proximal tibial resection for bone tumors. An analysis of function and outcome comparing allograft and prosthetic reconstructions. Clin Orthop 1994;303:116 – 27.

[16] Hornicek FJ, Mnaymneh W, Lackman MD, et al. Limb salvage with osteoarticular allografts after resection of proximal tibia bone tumors. Clin Orthop 1998;352: 179 – 85.

[17] Gebhardt MC, Roth YF, Mankin HJ. Osteoarticular allografts for reconstruction in the proximal part of the humerus after excision of a musculoskeletal tumor. J Bone Joint Surg Am 1990;72:334 – 45.

[18] Getty PJ, Peabody TD. Complications and functional outcomes of reconstruction with an osteoarticular allograft after intra-articular resection of the proximal aspect of the humerus. J Bone Joint Surg Am 1999; 81:1138 – 46.

[19] DeGroot H, Donati D, Di Liddo M, et al. The use of cement in osteoarticular allografts for proximal humeral bone tumors. Clin Orthop 2004;427:190 – 7.

[20] Kocher MS, Gebhardt MC, Manhin HJ. Reconstruction of the distal aspect of the radius with use of an osteoarticular allograft after excision of a skeletal tumor. J Bone Joint Surg Am 1998;80:407 – 19.

[21] Ayerza MA, Muscolo DL, Aponte-Tinao LA. Unicompartmental osteoarticular allografts of the knee: survival analysis and complications. Proceedings of the 72nd Annual Meeting of the American Academy of Orthopaedic Surgeons. Washington, DC: AAOS; 2005. p. 627.

[22] Weiner SD, Scarborough M, Vander Griend RA. Resection arthrodesis of the knee with an intercalary allograft. J Bone Joint Surg Am 1996;78:185 – 92.

[23] Donati D, Giacomini S, Gozzi E, et al. Allograft arthrodesis treatment of bone tumors: a two-center study. Clin Orthop 2002;400:217 – 24.

[24] Amitani A, Yamazaki T, Sonoda J, et al. Preservation of the knee joint in limb salvage of osteosarcoma in the proximal tibia. Int Orthop 1998;22:330 – 4.

[25] Canadell J, Forriol F, Cara JA. Removal of metaphy-

seal bone tumors with preservation of the epiphysis. Physeal distraction before excision. J Bone Joint Surg Br 1994;76:127 – 32.

[26] Kumta SM, Chow TC, Griffith J, et al. Classifying the location of osteosarcoma with reference to the epiphyseal plate helps determine the optimal skeletal resection in limb salvage procedure. Arch Orthop Trauma Surg 1999;119:327 – 31.

[27] Manfrini M, Gasbarrini A, Malaguti C, et al. Intraepiphyseal resection of the proximal tibia and its impact on lower limb growth. Clin Orthop 1999;358: 111 – 9.

[28] Muscolo DL, Ayerza MA, Aponte-Tinao LA, et al. Partial epiphyseal preservation and intercalary allograft reconstruction in high-grade metaphyseal osteosarcoma of the knee. J Bone Joint Surg Am 2004;86: 2686 – 93.

[29] Shinoara N, Sumida S, Masuda S. Bone allografts after segmental resection of tumors. Int Orthop 1990; 14:273 – 6.

[30] Tsuchiya H, Abdel-Wanis ME, Sakurakichi K, et al. Osteosarcoma around the knee. Intraepiphyseal excision and biological reconstruction with distraction osteogenesis. J Bone Joint Surg Br 2002;84:1162 – 6.

[31] Ortiz-Cruz EJ, Gebhardt MC, Jennings LC, et al. The results of transplantation of intercalary allografts after resection of tumors: a long- term follow-up study. J Bone Joint Surg Am 1997;79:97 – 106.

[32] Cara JA, Laclériga A, Cañadell J. Intercalary bone allografts: 23 tumor cases followed for 3 years. Acta Orthop Scand 1994;65:42 – 6.

[33] Muscolo DL, Ayerza MA, Aponte-Tinao LA, et al. Intercalary femur and tibia segmental allografts provide an acceptable alternative in reconstructing tumor resections. Clin Orthop 2004;426:97 – 102.

[34] Deijkers RL, Bloem RM, Hogendoorn PC, et al. Hemicortical allograft reconstruction after resection of low-grade malignant bone tumours. J Bone Joint Surg Br 2002;84:1009 – 14.

[35] Ayerza MA, Aponte-Tinao LA, Muscolo DL, et al. Combined fragmented and structural cortical allograft reconstruction after intralesional curettage of giant cell tumor of the distal femur. Orthopedics 2006, in press.

[36] Gitelis S, Piasecki P. Allograft prosthetic composite arthroplasty for osteosarcoma and other aggressive bone tumors. Clin Orthop 1991;270:197 – 201.

[37] Zehr RJ, Enneking WF, Scarborough MT. Allograftprosthesis composite versus megaprosthesis in proximal femoral reconstruction. Clin Orthop 1996;322: 207 – 23.

[38] Langlais F, Lambotte JC, Collin P, et al. Long-term results of allograft composite total hip prostheses for tumors. Clin Orthop 2003;414:197 – 211.

[39] Wilkins RM, Kelly CM. Revision of the failed distal femoral replacement to allograft prosthetic composite. Clin Orthop 2002;397:114 – 8.

ELSEVIER
SAUNDERS

Orthop Clin N Am 37 (2006) 75 – 84

ORTHOPEDIC
CLINICS
OF NORTH AMERICA

The Use of Prostheses in Skeletally Immature Patients

Adesegun Abudu, FRCS*, Robert Grimer, FRCS, Roger Tillman, FRCS,
Simon Carter, FRCS

Royal Orthopaedic Hospital, Bristol Road South, Birmingham B31 2AP, UK

The discovery of effective chemotherapy and the realization of the high functional and economic cost associated with amputation have led to the popularity of limb-preserving surgery in the treatment of patients who have bone sarcoma [1,2]. The challenge of preserving the limb of a skeletally immature patient with primary bone sarcoma includes maintenance of limb length after resection of one or more major growth plates and the need to use a durable reconstruction that can cope with the high functional and recreational demands of young patients, particularly now that most of the patients are expected to survive their disease because of the availability of effective chemotherapy.

The options for reconstruction of major bone defects after excision of primary bone sarcoma in children can be broadly classified as biologic, nonbiologic, or combined (biologic and nonbiologic). Biologic reconstructions using allografts or vascularized autogenous grafts have considerable theoretic attractions and are undoubtedly the best procedure for diaphyseal defects in upper and lower limbs. Biologic reconstructions do not work well in patients requiring osteoarticular reconstruction when preservation of joint motion is desirable and are even less successful in children in clinical practice [3–5]. The combination of allograft and prosthesis as a composite is an option, but the results of this type of reconstruction are similar to endoprosthetic replacement alone [6,7].

Nonbiologic reconstruction using a prosthesis has the advantages of allowing early weight bearing, having predictable function, having low risks of early

complications, and being readily available. The prostheses are expensive, however, and complications are expected to increase with time in surviving patients. Extendable prostheses allow maintenance of limb length in skeletally immature patients who require resection of one or more major growth plates for the treatment of their tumors. This article aims to describe the development, indications, and clinical results of using extendable prostheses for limb reconstruction in the skeletally immature patient.

Indication for extendable prostheses

Appositional and longitudinal bone growth is expected in the immature skeleton. Primary malignant bone tumors in children predominantly occur in the metaphyseal region close to the growth plate such that sacrifice of a major physis is often necessary when the tumor is excised. Furthermore, children who have primary bone sarcoma often require chemotherapy, and this has a suppressive effect on bone growth [8,9]. The amount of bone growth that can be expected from each growth plate has been estimated. Generally, about 60% to 70% of lower-limb growth occurs around the knee (distal femur and proximal tibia physes) and about 80% of total growth of the humerus occurs in the proximal physis of the humerus [10–12]. Cool and colleagues [13] showed that the growth of the remaining physis of the operated limb is further delayed after limb-preserving surgery.

The severity of limb-length discrepancy after excision of a major growth plate depends on the patient's bone age estimated from plain radiographs

* Corresponding author.
E-mail address: seggy.abudu@roh.nhs.uk (A. Abudu).

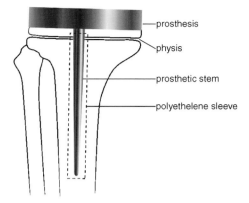

Fig. 1. Schematic illustration of a sliding component in the proximal tibia. The proximal tibial physis is preserved and the uncemented smooth prosthesis slides within the polyethelene sleeve as the physis grows.

of the hands according to the radiologic atlas of Greulich and Pyle [14] at the time of surgery. Younger patients are expected to have larger bone discrepancy. It is desirable to restore limb length whenever possible because significant leg-length discrepancy results in gait abnormalities, leg pain, and back pain; in the upper limb, a short arm is cosmetically embarrassing [15].

Extendable prostheses are required when the estimated leg-length discrepancy at skeletal maturity is more than 3 cm or when the arm-length discrepancy is more than 5 cm. When the estimated arm-length discrepancy is less than 5 cm, a prostheses made up to 2 to 3 cm longer can be inserted in patients requiring proximal humeral or total humeral prostheses such that the operated upper limb is initially longer but the opposite limb will soon catch up: at skeletal maturity, the child may have an equal length or a slightly shorter upper limb. The main problem with slight arm-length discrepancy is cosmetic, and problems with bimanual tasks occur only when there is a large difference [16].

In the lower limbs, patients who have less than 3 cm of estimated leg-length discrepancy can be treated with conventional "adult-type" prostheses made longer by up to 1.5 cm, and a "sliding" prosthetic component can be used across the remaining open physis. The sliding component is an uncemented smooth component placed within a plastic sleeve through a centrally made canal in the remaining preserved physis. This technique, in principle, allows this component to slide inside the bone as the remaining open physis grows (Fig. 1). The amount of the growth plate destroyed by insertion of the

sliding component is not more than 13% in the distal femur and proximal tibia, and there is no correlation between the surface areas destroyed and continued growth of the physes [17–19]. The physes grow without any deformity but at a slower rate, achieving about 80% of normal growth in the proximal tibia and about 60% of normal growth in the distal femur compared with the contralateral limb [17–19].

Girls older than 11 years or boys older than 13 years rarely require extendable prostheses because the estimated growth discrepancy after these ages is less than 3 cm. In these cases, adult-type prostheses can be made longer by up to 1.5 cm and combined with a sliding component across the remaining physis.

Development and evolution of extendable prostheses

The authors' center began to use extendable prostheses in children about 30 years ago. The first design in 1976 consisted of a titanium alloy shaft and stem and a delrin hemiknee, and the extension device used a worm drive mechanism. The gearing mechanism was unreliable, however, and a new extension mechanism was devised in 1982 that used ball bearings, whereby the bearings were forced through a porthole in the prosthesis to jack out the pusher and thereby extend the prosthesis (Fig. 2). This prosthesis

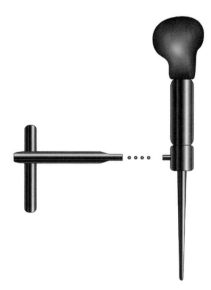

Fig. 2. Schematic illustration of an earlier type of extendible endoprosthesis of the proximal humerus that used ball bearings as an extension mechanism of the prosthesis.

was more successful but still proved unreliable due to fracture of the ball bearing and jamming of the extension port. This design was replaced in 1988 with a newer type of extension mechanism that used C-collars (Fig. 3). The C-collar was essentially a modular insert placed between the body and stem components of the prosthesis. The C-collars are replaced with longer ones at intervals to gain length. This type of extension mechanism was more successful and used until 1993, but its major disadvantages were that patients required extensive wound incisions at least 2 cm longer than the collar to be inserted (with consequent prolonged hospital stay), there was increased risk of infection and scarring, and sudden failure occasionally occurred by displacement of the collar. The C-collar design was replaced in 1993 with a minimally invasive extension mechanism that used a customized Allen screwdriver (Fig. 4). This design was revolutionary in that it allowed the lengthening to be performed percutaneously as a day procedure through a stab incision under image intensification with reduced risk of infection. Patients, however, still required general anesthesia and, rarely, experienced sudden unplanned length-

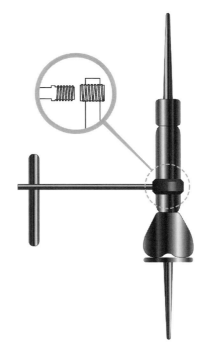

Fig. 4. Schematic illustration of a minimally invasive extendable endoprosthesis of the distal femur, whereby a customized Allen screwdriver is used as extension mechanism. The screwdriver is inserted through a stab incision. This mechanism has largely been replaced by noninvasive mechanisms, but the authors still use it in patients who may require MRI for future follow-up.

ening or shortening. This design is still in use but has largely been replaced by noninvasive extendable prostheses in which electromagnetic energy is used to distract the lengthening mechanism. This noninvasive extendable prosthesis is certainly the way forward because it does not require anesthesia or an operative procedure and, hence, the risk of infection is reduced. The disadvantage of the noninvasive extendible prosthesis is that it cannot be used uncemented because forceful impaction of the prosthesis damages the magnetic lengthening device. In addition, patients who have noninvasive extendible prostheses are unable to have MRI scans because of the magnetic lengthening device and require longer bone resection to achieve the same length of extension compared with minimally invasive prostheses.

All of the prostheses were custom-made and manufactured by Stanmore Implant Worldwide, Department of Biomedical Engineering, Institute of Orthopaedics, Stanmore, England, UK [20].

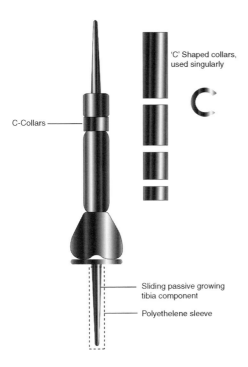

'C' Shaped collars, used singularly

C-Collars

Sliding passive growing tibia component

Polyethelene sleeve

Fig. 3. Schematic illustration of an extendable endoprosthesis of the distal femur with C-collars used as the extension mechanism. The modular C-collars are changed at intervals to longer collars to gain length.

Clinical results and complications of extendable prostheses

Several authors have reported good clinical outcomes with the use of extendable prostheses in children, but complications remain a major concern and tend to increase with time [16,17,21–24]. The authors' experience of using extendable endoprostheses spans 3 decades. The authors have performed 180 extendable prostheses in 176 patients between 1976 and 2005 (Fig. 5). Five patients presented with pathologic fracture. The mean follow-up from the date of surgery to date of last review or death was 96 months (range, 7–263 months) for all patients. One hundred seventeen patients are still alive at a median follow-up of 11 years (range, 1–22 years). The mean age of the patients treated at the time of surgery was 9.6 years (range, 2–15 years). One hundred thirty-five patients (77%) had reached skeletal maturity at the time of last follow-up or before death from disease.

The predominant diagnoses were osteosarcoma (131 patients) and Ewing's sarcoma (34 patients).

The prostheses were distal femur (91), proximal tibia (42), proximal humerus (20), total humerus (6), total femur (6), and proximal femur (11).

Complications were frequent, occurring in 85 patients (48%), and included infection, local recurrence, aseptic loosening, joint stiffness, periprosthetic fracture, hip joint sublxation, and outgrowing of prostheses.

Infection

Deep prosthetic infection is a major concern in children who have extendable prostheses because of the need for multiple operative procedures. The cumulative risk of infection in the authors' series was 21% at 10 years (Figs. 6 and 7). The infections often follow surgical procedures such as lengthening, rebushing, or revision and are more common after open operations than percutaneous procedures. The risk of infection varies in different sites, with the proximal tibia being the most common site because of its relatively superficial location and poor soft tissue cover. The risk of infection after extendable proximal tibial endoprosthesis is 5% per open lengthening procedure, and the cumulative risk of infection is 68% at 10 years in the tibia compared with 3% in the femur and 2% in the humerus per open lengthening procedure. Routine use of a gastrocnemius flap to improve soft tissue cover and to reconstruct the

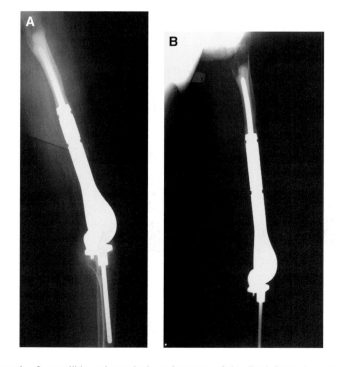

Fig. 5. (*A*) Plain radiograph of extendible endoprosthetic replacement of the distal femur in an 8-year-old boy. (*B*) Later radiograph of the same patient illustrating the amount of growth achieved using C-collars.

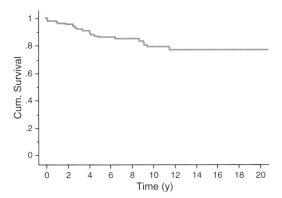

Fig. 6. Cumulative risk of infection after extendble endoprosthesis in all skeletally immature patients.

knee extensor mechanism has helped to significantly reduce infection risk after tibial prostheses; however, infection remains a major problem [25,26]. Two-stage revision surgery of infected prostheses is successful in about 70% of cases [27].

Other investigators have identified infection as a major problem in children who have extendable endoprostheses, with rates of between 15% and 23% [21,23,24]. The authors' experience is that infection risk due to minimally invasive lengthening is low compared with open procedures. Prosthetic infection developed in 7 of 84 patients (8%) who received minimally invasive prostheses, whereas 25 of 92 patients (27%) who received earlier types of prostheses requiring open lengthening developed infection. The authors anticipate that the use of noninvasive extendable endoprostheses will reduce the number of surgical procedures in these children and lead to further reduction of infection risk. Because the children are likely to require other procedures unrelated to lengthening, however, prosthetic infection is unlikely to be eradicated in children who have extendable endoprostheses. A recent report of early experience of noninvasive lengthening by Gitelis and colleagues [28] reported an infection risk of 6% at an average follow-up of 24 months in 18 patients.

Local recurrence

Local recurrence is mainly related to adequacy of surgery and response to preoperative chemotherapy [29–31]. Children undergoing any form of limb-preserving surgery have increased risk of local recurrence compared with those who undergo amputation [29–31]. Survival of the patients, however, is similar irrespective of the method of treatment (ie, limb preservation or amputation) [32,33].

Local recurrence occurred in 25 patients (14%) at a median time of 19 months (range, 6–114 months). It should be noted that the period of study under review was about 30 years, during which time significant advances occurred in imaging, chemotherapy, and surgical expertise. The rate of local

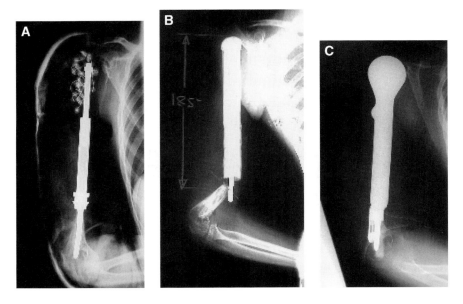

Fig. 7. (*A*) Infected extendable endoprosthesis of the proximal humerus. (*B*, *C*) Two-stage revision is usually successful.

recurrence in this study is broadly similar to the risk reported in other major series of limb-preserving surgery, whether in adults or children [30,31]. The treatment of local recurrence was amputation in 11 patients and excision in 14 patients. Nine of the patients who developed local recurrence are currently alive and free of disease, 2 are alive with disease, and 14 died of disease. Development of local recurrence was associated with significantly worse survival, with a cumulative survival rate of only 8% at 5 years.

Stiffness

Joint stiffness is sometimes a problem after extendable endoprosthesis around the knee. This complication occurred in 25 patients (14%) in the authors' series and was seen only in patients who had prostheses around the knee. Thirteen of the patients who experienced stiffness had received extendable proximal tibia prostheses and 12 had received distal femur prostheses. The risk of stiffness after extendable proximal tibial and distal femur endoprosthesis is 31% and 13%, respectively. The risk factors for developing stiffness include scarring associated with open operations for lengthening or revision surgery and excessive lengthening. The authors recommend small lengthening of about 6 mm each time, although in carefully selected patients, lengthening up to 10 mm may be performed. In addition, physiotherapy is mandatory to maintain joint motion after lengthening, and further lengthening should be delayed for a period of at least 6 weeks to prevent stiffness. Joint stiffness may be an early sign of low-grade prosthetic infection, and patients who have stiffness should be appropriately investigated with serum inflammatory markers and aspiration of the prostheses to exclude infection.

Stiffness of the knee after extendable prostheses can often be treated with manipulation under anesthesia, serial casting, and intensive physiotherapy. Surgical exploration and release of scar tissues is necessary only in a few recalcitrant cases unresponsive to nonsurgical treatment.

Periprosthetic and implant fracture

Children who require extendable endoprostheses are expected to place great demands on their prostheses because of their young age and sporting and occupational aspirations in the survivors. It is advisable to inform the patients to avoid impact and contact sports, although the authors' experience is that such advice is not often heeded. Some of the authors' patients play soccer, tennis, and badminton; hence, fracture of the implant or the bones around implants is a major concern. The risk of fracturing is about 8% in the authors' series. Fourteen patients developed fracture of the implant or the bone by the time of last follow-up. All of the fractures were in prostheses in the lower limbs, including distal femur replacement in 9 patients, proximal tibia replacement in 4, and midfemur replacement in 1. Eight patients had fracture of the prostheses and 6 had bony fractures. The median time from surgery to fracture was 69 months (range, 4–191 months).

Periprosthetic fracture is usually associated with the sliding component, which is not secured in any way to the bone to allow continued growth of the physis across the joint (Fig. 8). Nonoperative treatment of the fractures is often unsuccessful because the primary cause of the fracture is lack of fixation of the sliding component. Revision surgery to a longer stem, cemented prosthesis is recommended. Fracture may also occur in patients who have aseptic loosening, but this complication has not been seen in the authors' series. Implant fracture is almost certainly related to fatigue, and improved implant metallurgy may help to decrease its occurrence. The authors have not seen any implant fractures in the 85 patients treated with extendable prostheses at their center in the last 12 years. Because the upper limb is not a weight-bearing limb, fracture of bones or an implant at this site is rare.

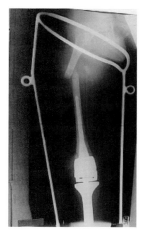

Fig. 8. Periprosthetic fracture around an extendable endoprosthesis is a problem in the long-term. Treatment with fracture fixation or revision to another prosthesis with a longer stem is usually successful.

Joint subluxation

Subluxation of the hip and shoulder joint is an area of concern in young patients who undergo extendable endoprosthesis. Although extendable prostheses can correct limb-length discrepancy, delayed growth of the acetabulum and glenoid is not easy to correct. This area has been one of major concern, particularly in patients who undergo such operations before age 7 years. Delayed acetabular growth due to combination of loss of normal femoral head after proximal femur replacement invariably leads to acetabular dysplasia. Subsequent lengthening of the prosthesis only accentuates the subluxation. Replacement of the acetabulum in children who have open triradiate cartilage is not advisable. When acetabular dysplasia and hip subluxation occur, patients often present with pain and limitation of activity, which usually require further intervention. The authors have performed pelvic osteotomy and even used allografts to reconstruct the acetabulum (Fig. 9) but without success. It appears that the only reliable treatment for this condition is acetabular replacement when the child reaches skeletal maturity or when the triradiate cartilage has closed (Fig. 10). This methodology has been the authors' recent policy (using an uncemented acetabular component), and although early experience has been good, no long-term follow-up is available.

Some investigators advise against the use of extendable proximal humeral prostheses because they consider that lengthening of the humeral prosthesis

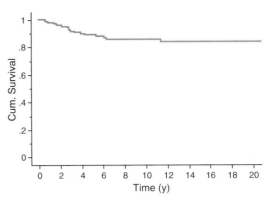

Fig. 10. Long-term cumulative risk of amputation for any reason in all patients treated with extendable endoprostheses.

only results in shoulder subluxation without lengthening of the arm [34]. Symptomatic subluxation of the shoulder, however, is uncommon, and satisfactory arm lengthening can be achieved in the authors' experience [16]. This result is probably because of the use of a restraining mesh placed around the humeral head. The authors try to preserve the acromion and coracoacromial ligament whenever possible to prevent subluxation; however, a slight amount of proximal subluxation after lengthening inevitably occurs in most patients because the rotator cuff has been excised but the prostheses abuts superiorly against the acromion and the coracoacromial ligament. When subluxation of the shoulder becomes symptomatic, it is important to avoid further lengthening if possible because the consequence of a slightly shortened upper limb is not as great as a shortened lower limb. For patients who have significant symptoms, the authors have found the use of a constrained glenoid implant to be a reliable way of treating such symptomatic subluxation of the shoulder.

Outgrowing extendable endoprostheses

Very young children requiring extendable endoprostheses and who survive their sarcomas are likely to outgrow the maximum length of extension that can be incorporated in their prostheses. The amount of extension built into an extendable prosthesis depends on the length of the prosthesis, which in turn is dependent on the amount of bone resection and the total length of the child's bone. Young children under age 7 years have short bones and need a smaller length of bone resection, although the percentage of bone resected may be similar to or larger than that in

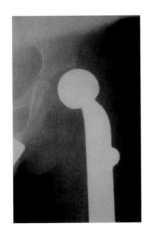

Fig. 9. Subluxation of the hip joint in young children who have proximal femur endoprostheses mostly occurs in children who undergo surgery before age 7 years. Allograft or pelvic osteotomy has not been successful in preventing this complication.

adults. The maximum amount of lengthening that can be built into an extendable prosthesis is 120 mm; hence, a young child may require an exchange of the prosthesis to a new one when the maximum prosthetic extension is reached and further growth is anticipated.

Aseptic loosening

It is inevitable that young children who have extendable endoprostheses will develop aseptic loosening. This complication is due to a combination of circumferential or appositional bone growth and mechanical factors. Appositional bone growth results in widening of the bone and the intramedullary canal, with consequent loosening of the prosthesis. Children also place much greater demands on their prostheses. Revision for aseptic loosening is usually straightforward, but efforts are required to minimize this problem. Aseptic loosening is more common after extendable endoprosthesis in the proximal tibia and distal femur than in the humerus and proximal femur [16,17,35–37]. Young patients requiring more than 60% bone resection in the proximal tibia or the distal femur have the worst prognosis for aseptic loosening [38]. It is possible that the use of uncemented prostheses will reduce the risk of aseptic loosening, but clinical outcome studies are still awaited [39]. The addition of hydroxyapatite-coated collars at the host bone–prosthesis interface may result in improved longevity of cemented implants. The authors' experience is that cemented prostheses with hydroxyapatite collars have improved longevity compared with those without hydroxyapatite collars, with only one aseptic loosening seen in about 500 patients treated with such prostheses in the last 10 years [40].

Conversion of an extendable prosthesis to an adult-type prosthesis is performed when the child reaches skeletal maturity and there is aseptic loosening. The authors consider such conversion to an adult-type endoprosthesis as part of the treatment plan for any skeletally immature child who has an extendable prosthesis.

Function and quality of life after extendable prosthesis

Several investigators have reported good to excellent functional results after extendable endoprostheses, with functional scores far superior to those of amputation and the functional outcome similar to that reported for adult patients [16,17, 21–24,28,41,42]. Prosthetic reconstruction is well received emotionally and cosmetically by patients and their parents. Despite the high rates of complications and multiple operations, the children have a favorable quality of life [43]. The availability of noninvasive endoprostheses, leading to fewer operative interventions, is anticipated to result in improved functional scores.

Long-term risk of amputation after extendable endoprosthesis

Nineteen patients (11%) needed amputations because of local recurrence (11) and infection (8). The cumulative risk of amputation for any reason was 15% at 20 years (see Fig. 10).

Summary

Endoprosthetic reconstruction in children is fraught with several problems, but satisfactory functional limbs can be maintained in the long-term. An extendable prosthesis allows maintenance of limb length and is cosmetically and emotionally acceptable to patients and their parents. Complications include infection, local recurrence, aseptic loosening, joint stiffness, subluxation, periprosthetic fracture, and outgrowing the prosthesis. The risk of amputation for treatment of complications is low in the long-term. The advent of noninvasive extendable prostheses is expected to significantly reduce the problems associated with multiple operations and infection. Fixation of a hydroxyapatite collar to the host bone to prevent aseptic loosening is beneficial.

Patients and their parents need to be made aware of the likely course of events before embarking on extendable endoprosthetic replacement, and alternative forms of treatment should be discussed. Amputation offers excellent local control, but function is poor, emotional and economic cost to the patient is high, and overgrowth of the stump may occur. Rotationplasty is a well-established surgical alternative for children who have tumors in the femur and proximal tibia, but most patients and parents find it unacceptable in many communities, and significant early and late complications also occur [44–46].

References

[1] Renard AJ, Veth RP, Schreuder HW, et al. Function and complications after ablative and limb salvage therapy in lower extremity sarcoma of bone. J Surg Oncol 2000;73:198–205.

[2] Cara JA, Canadell J. Limb salvage for malignant bone tumours in young children. J Pediatr Orthop 1994;14: 112–8.

[3] Alman BA, De Bari A, Krajbich JI. Massive allografts in the treatment of osteosarcoma and Ewing's sarcoma in children and adolescent. J Bone Joint Surg Am 1995;77:54–64.

[4] Brien EW, Terek RM, Healy JH, et al. Allograft reconstruction after proximal tibial resection for bone tumours. An analysis of function and outcome comparing allograft and prosthetic reconstruction. Clin Orthop Relat Res 1994;303:116–27.

[5] Rodl RW, Ozaki T, Hoffman C, et al. Osteoarticular allograft in surgery for high-grade malignant tumours of bone. J Bone Joint Surg Br 2000;82:1006–10.

[6] Zehr RJ, Enneking WF, Scarborough MT. Allograft-prosthesis composite versus megaprosthesis in proximal femur reconstructions. Clin Orthop Relat Res 1996;322:207–23.

[7] McGovern BM, Davis AM, Gross AE, et al. Evaluation of allograft-prosthesis composite technique for proximal femur reconstruction after resection of a primary bone tumour. Can J Surg 1999;42:37–45.

[8] Glasser DB, Duane K, Lane JM, et al. The effect of chemotherapy on growth in the skeletally immature individual. Clin Orthop 1991;262:93–100.

[9] Cool WP, Grimer RJ, Carter SR, et al. Longitudinal growth following treatment for osteosarcoma. Sarcoma 1998;2:115–9.

[10] Exner UG. Wachstum der unteren Extremität. In: Exner UG, editor. Normalwerte in der Kinderorthopädie. Stuttgart, Germany: Georg Thieme Verlag; 1990. p. 68–78 [in German].

[11] Bisgard JD, Bisgard ME. Longitudinal growth of long bones. Arch Surg 1935;31:568–78.

[12] Pritchett JW. Growth plate activity in the upper extremity. Clin Ortho and Relat Res 1991;268:235–42.

[13] Cool WP, Carter SR, Grimer RJ, et al. Growth after extendible endoprosthetic replacement in the distal femur. J Bone Joint Surg Br 1997;79:938–42.

[14] Greulich WW, Pyle SI. Radiographic atlas of skeletal development of the hand and wrist. 2nd edition. Stanford (CA): Stanford University Press; 1959.

[15] Song KM, Halliday SE, Little DG. The effect of limb length on gait. J Bone Joint Surg Am 1997;79:1690–8.

[16] Ayoub KS, Fiorenza F, Grimer RJ, et al. Extensible endoprostheses of the humerus after resection of bone tumours. J Bone Joint Surg Br 1999;81:495–500.

[17] Grimer RJ, Belthur M, Carter SR, et al. Extendible replacements of the proximal tibia for bone tumours. J Bone Joint Surg Br 2000;82:255–60.

[18] Cool WP, Carter SR, Grimer RJ, et al. Growth after extendible endoprosthetic replacement in the distal femur. J Bone Joint Surg Br 1997;79:938–42.

[19] Cool WP, Grimer RJ, Carter SR, et al. Passive growth at the sliding component following endoprosthetic replacement in skeletally immature children with primary bone tumour around the knee. J Bone Joint Surg Br 1996;78(Suppl 1):33.

[20] Scales JT, Sneath RS, Wright KWJ. Design and clinical use of extending prostheses. In: Enneking WF, editor. Limb salvage in musculoskeletal oncology. New York: Churchill Livingstone; 1987. p. 52–61.

[21] Kenan S, Lewis MM. Limb salvage in pediatric surgery: the use of extendable prostheses. Orthop Clin North Am 1991;22:121–31.

[22] Eckardt JJ, Safran MR, Eilber FR, et al. Expandable endoprosthetic reconstruction of the skeletally immature after malignant bone tumour resection. Clin Orthop Relat Res 1993;297:188–202.

[23] Delepine G, Delepine N, Desbois JC, et al. Expanding prostheses in conservative surgery for lower limb sarcoma. Int Orthop 1998;22:27–31.

[24] Schiller C, Windhager R, Fellinger EJ, et al. Extendable tumour endoprostheses for the leg in children. J Bone Joint Surg Br 1995;77:608–14.

[25] Grimer RJ, Shewell PC, Carter SR, et al. Endoprosthetic replacement of the proximal tibia. J Bone Joint Surg Br 1999;81:488–94.

[26] Grimer RJ, Ratcliffe P, Carter SR, et al. Reduction of infection of proximal tibia endoprostheses. In: Brown KLB, editor. Complications of limb salvage: prevention, management and outcome. Montreal, Canada: International Society of Limb Salvage; 1991. p. 331.

[27] Jeys LM, Grimer RJ, Carter SR, et al. Peri-prosthetic infection in patients treated for an orthopaedic oncological condition. J Bone Joint Surg Am 2005;87: 842–9.

[28] Gitelis S, Neel MD, Wilkins RM, et al. The use of a closed expandable prosthesis for paediatric sarcomas. Chir Organi Mov 2003;88:327–33.

[29] Grimer RJ, Taminiau AM, Cannon SR. Surgical subcommittee on behalf of the European Osteosarcoma Intergroup. Surgical outcomes in osteosarcoma. J Bone Joint Surg Br 2002;84:395–400.

[30] Tsuchiya H, Tomita K. Prognosis of osteosarcoma treated by limb salvage surgery: the ten-year intergroup study in Japan. Jpn L Clin Oncol 1992;22:347–53.

[31] Bacci G, Ferrari S, Mecuri M, et al. Predictive factors for local recurrence in osteosarcoma: 540 patients who have extremity tumours followed for minimum 2.5 years after neoadjuvant chemotherapy. Acta Orthop Scand 1998;69:230–6.

[32] Simon MA, Aschiliman MA, Thomas N, et al. Limb salvage treatment versus amputation for osteosarcoma of the distal end of the femur. J Bone Joint Surg Am 1986;68:1331–7.

[33] Rougraff BT, Simon MA, Kneist JS, et al. Limb salvage compared with amputation for osteosarcoma of the distal end of the femur. J Bone Joint Surg Am 1994;76:649–56.

[34] Lavy CBD, Briggs TWR. Failure of growing endoprosthetic replacement of the humerus. J Bone Joint Surg Br 1992;74:626.

[35] Schindler OS, Cannon SR, Briggs TW, et al. Stanmore custom-made extendible distal femur replacements. Clinical experience in children with primary malignant bone tumours. J Bone Joint Surg Br 1997;79:927–37.

[36] Unwin PS, Walker PS. Extendible endoprostheses for the skeletally immature. Clin Orthop Relat Res 1996; 322:179–93.

[37] Belthur M, Suneja R, Grimer RJ, et al. Extensible endoprostheses for bone tumours of the proximal femur in children. J Pediatr Orthop 2003;23:230–5.

[38] Unwin PS, Cannon SR, Grimer RJ, et al. Aspetic loosening in cemented custom-made prosthetic replacements for bone tumours of the lower limb. J Bone Joint Surg Br 1996;78:5–13.

[39] Blunn GW, Briggs TW, Cannon SR, et al. Cementless fixation for primary segmental bone tumour endoprostheses. Clin Orthop Relat Res 2000;372: 223–30.

[40] Unwin PS, Walker PS, Briggs TW, et al. Rotating hinged, hydroxyapatite coated verses fixed hinged, uncoated distal femoral replacemements. A study of 402 cases. Presented at the Tenth International Symposium on Limb Salvage. Cairns, Australia, April 1999.

[41] Schindler OS, Cannon SR, Briggs TWR, et al. Use of extendable total femoral replacements in children with malignant bone tumours. Clin Orthop Relat Res 1998; 357:157–70.

[42] Krepler P, Dominkus M, Toma CD, et al. Endoprosthesis management of the extremities of children after resection of primary malignant bone tumours. Orthopade 2003;32:1013–9.

[43] Eiser C, Cool P, Grimer RJ, et al. Quality of life in children following treatment for a malignant primary bone tumour around the knee. Sarcoma 1997; 1:39–45.

[44] Gottsauner-Wolf F, Kotx R, Knahr K, et al. Rotationplasty for limb salvage in the treatment of malignant tumours at the knee. A follow-up study of seventy patients. J Bone Joint Surg Am 1991;73:1365–75.

[45] Rodl RW, Pohlmann U, Gosheger G, et al. Rotationplasty—quality of life after 10 years in 22 patients. Acta Orthop Scand 2002;73:85–8.

[46] Winklemann WW. Type-B-IIIa hip rotationplasty: an alternative operation for the treatment of malignant tumours of the femur in early childhood. J Bone Joint Surg Am 2000;82:814–28.

ELSEVIER
SAUNDERS

Orthop Clin N Am 37 (2006) 85 – 97

ORTHOPEDIC
CLINICS
OF NORTH AMERICA

Pelvic Reconstruction Techniques

Ronald Hugate, Jr, MD[a], Franklin H. Sim, MD[b],*

[a]Colorado Limb Consultants, 1601 East 19th Avenue, Suite 3300, Denver, CO 80218, USA
[b]Department of Orthopedic Surgery, Division of Orthopedic Oncology, Mayo Clinic, 200 First Street SW,
Rochester MN 55905, USA

Partial resection of the pelvis or sacrum is an uncommon procedure, typically performed in the setting of tumors, severe infections, or trauma. The resultant defects, depending on the size and location, may cause significant postoperative morbidity or functional impairment. It is therefore essential that the surgeon be aware of all reconstructive options available and implement the most appropriate option for each individual patient. The purpose of this article is to review the functional consequences of the various pelvic resections and discuss the options available for reconstruction.

Types of resections

Pelvic and sacral resections vary widely in size and shape, depending on the extent, nature, and location of the lesions being addressed. Consequently, the reconstructive options are variable as well. In an effort to improve the dialogue among institutions with regard to these resections (and their subsequent reconstructive options), Enneking and Dunham [1] proposed a classification scheme for description of the various subtypes of pelvic resections in 1978. This classification scheme is still relevant today and is frequently referred to in the literature. For the purposes of this article, the authors refer to this clas-

sification scheme, with a brief description provided in this section (Fig. 1).

Pelvic

Type I resections are those that involve all or part of the ilium, sparing the acetabulum (Fig. 2). The ilium serves two primary functions: First, it provides continuity between the acetabulum and the central skeleton by means of the sacroiliac articulation. Second, it provides a major soft tissue attachment site for the abdominal, gluteal, pelvic floor, rectus femoris, sartorius, and the iliacus muscles within the pelvis. Variations within this subset of resections include complete removal of the ilium and removal of only a small portion (Fig. 3). The biomechanical consequences vary a good deal within this spectrum. Certainly, complete removal of the ilium "disconnects" the acetabulum from the ipsilateral sacroiliac joint and may cause significant destabilization of the remaining segment, because it now hinges on the pubic symphysis. Partial resection of the iliac wing, by contrast, is a much less morbid procedure if continuity is maintained between the acetabulum and the axial skeleton. Resection of the ilium is referred to as type I-A when it involves removal of the gluteal musculature. Type I-S resections are those that involve a portion of the sacrum; they are also sometimes referred to as "extended hemipelvectomies."

Type II pelvic resections are those that involve resection of the periacetabular region of the pelvis. Typically, the three bony cuts for this resection are made superior to the dome of the acetabulum and at the lateral extents of the ischial and pubic rami. This is

* Corresponding author.
E-mail address: sim.franklin@mayo.edu (F.H. Sim).

0030-5898/06/$ – see front matter © 2005 Elsevier Inc. All rights reserved.
doi:10.1016/j.ocl.2005.08.006

orthopedic.theclinics.com

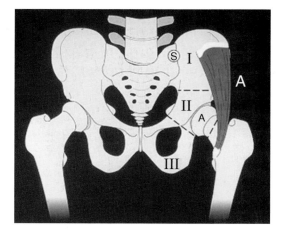

Fig. 1. Subtypes of pelvic resections as described by En-neking and Dunham in 1978.

perhaps the most debilitating form of pelvic resection, because the acetabulum and frequently the femoral head must be resected. Type II resections that involve the femoral head are referred to as type II-A resections. With the hip joint removed, the surgeon must address difficult issues, such as functionality, preservation of limb length, and hip stability.

Type III resections involve the ischiopubic region of the pelvis (medial to the acetabulum and lateral to the symphysis pubis). The ischiopubic region of the pelvis acts primarily to complete the ring of the pelvis, adding to its intrinsic structural stability. In addition, the rectus abdominis, hamstring, obturator, and adductor muscle groups all use this region as their bony anchor points. Hence patients experience weakness in these muscle groups following resection. One must also frequently sacrifice the obturator nerve as it courses through the obturator foramen, further causing dysfunction of the adductor group. Type III resections are generally well tolerated from a structural standpoint, because the acetabuli remain in continuity with the axial skeleton.

Sacral

Partial or complete sacral resections are referred to as type IV pelvic resections. Again, there are a number of variations within this subgroup. These resections may generally be referred to as transverse, sagittal, or combined partial sacrectomies (Fig. 4). Many lesions abut or invade the sacroiliac joint medially and may require that a partial sagittal hemisacrectomy be performed to gain a margin, along with the pelvic resection.

When should external hemipelvectomy be considered?

Although limb-sparing procedures may be undertaken safely in most clinical scenarios, there are times when external hemipelvectomy should be considered the treatment of choice. The decision is often difficult, with complex factors such as functionality, body image, and emotional acceptance all playing a role. In general, if a partial pelvic resection does not allow for safe margins about the lesion, or if the consequences of extirpation of the lesion are such that the residual limb is essentially functionless, external hemipelvectomy should be strongly considered. Special attention should be paid to preoperative imaging and physical examination to help assess the relationship of the lesion to the lumbo-sacral plexus, the femoral neurovascular bundle, and the hip joint. As a general rule, if any two of these three structures must be resected along with the lesion, the functional outcome with limb-sparing surgery is considered poor. In these cases, one should strongly consider external hemipelvectomy. This decision should be made only after careful consideration of the issues by both the surgeon and the patient.

When is reconstruction necessary?

Pelvis

Once partial pelvic resection is chosen as the most appropriate treatment for a given lesion, careful thought should be given to whether reconstruction is necessary. Although reconstruction may afford the patient substantial functional benefits, these must be weighed against the potential added complications,

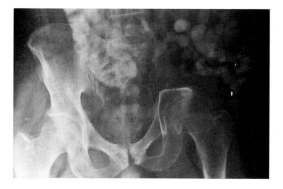

Fig. 2. A complete type I pelvic resection dissociates the acetabulum from the ipsilateral sacro-iliac joint. Note the pelvis discontinuity created by the resection.

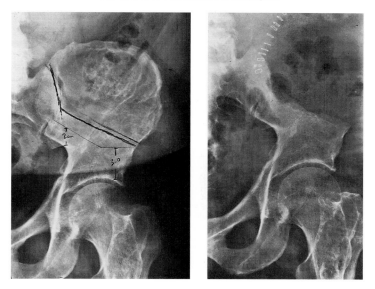

Fig. 3. Partial type I pelvic resection. Note that mechanical continuity is maintained with the sacrum.

operating time, blood loss, increased risk of infection, and so forth that can be part of the reconstruction process.

The main function of the pelvis is to provide bony continuity between the lower extremities and the central skeleton by means of articulations at the hip joints and sacroiliac joints. The pelvis also protects the pelvic contents and serves as the musculotendinous attachment point for a variety of muscle groups. Pelvic reconstruction following resection should be considered when one of two structural conditions exists: (1) there is loss of pelvic bony continuity between the acetabulum and the sacrum (ie, complete type I, I-A, or I-S resections) such that force cannot be transmitted from the lower extremity to the axial skeleton via the pelvis; or (2) the acetabulum is resected (ie, type II, II-A resections). Partial type I resections (when the pelvic ring remains in continuity) and complete type III resections typically do not require reconstruction. Deciding on the type of reconstruction to perform is a complex process informed by a number of factors.

Sacrum

The sacrum functions to transmit force between the lower limbs and the vertebral column and to protect neural elements (sacral nerve roots and thecal sac). The sacroiliac articulation is normally stabilized by a number of factors. The wedge-shaped bone is positioned between the two iliac wings. This arrangement confers intrinsic stability against inferior migration of the sacrum. The sacroiliac joint also has an irregular lining and therefore forms broad, interlocking surfaces with the ilium, which effectively resist motion. In addition, the strong sacroiliac, sacrotuberous, sacrospinous, and lumbo-sacral ligaments play an important role in the stabilization. These are among the strongest ligaments in the body. The combination of these factors renders the spinopelvic segment especially stable.

Patients who undergo complete sacrectomy generally require reconstruction. Without the sacrum, the ability to transmit forces from the lower extremities to the axial skeleton is gone. Conversely, the central skeleton no longer has a support and is therefore free to translate, constrained only nominally by soft tissues. The translation may be significant and may cause problems with pain or with mechanical kinking of blood vessels or viscera when moving from a supine to an upright position (Fig. 5). Having a flail central skeleton also precludes ambulation. For these reasons, iliolumbar arthrodesis is recommended in this setting.

The degree of need for sacral reconstruction following partial sacrectomy varies with the type of resection. If there is complete unilateral loss of the sacrum (sagittal hemisacrectomy), then reconstruction is indicated to reconstitute the pelvic ring. Transverse partial sacrectomies of the distal sacrum are well tolerated from a structural standpoint. The precise quantity of sacrum that may be amputated while maintaining mechanical stability is not clear based on the current literature.

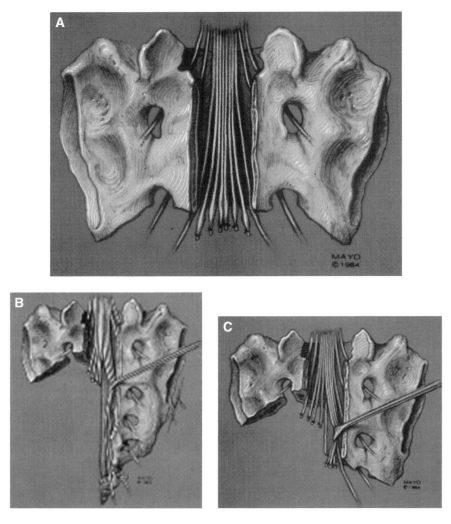

Fig. 4. (*A*) Transverse partial sacrectomy, (*B*) sagittal hemisacrectomy, and (*C*) combined type. (*Courtesy of* Mayo Foundation, Rochester, MN; with permission.)

The biomechanical consequences of transverse partial sacrectomies are poorly understood. Resection of the spinopelvic segment may require reconstruction using complex methods that involve iliolumbar arthrodesis. Such a reconstruction may add significant complexity and morbidity to sacral resection alone. Transverse hemisacrectomy below the S2 foramina and nerve root typically would not involve resection of the sacroiliac joints and would have minimal effect on stability. Transverse hemisacrectomies involving the S2 and S1 sacral bodies are not as well understood. Gunterberg and colleagues [2] studied sacropelvic biomechanics. Based on the data available at the time, Gunterberg concluded that transverse osteotomies, even involving a small portion of the sacral ala, could allow for early weight bearing postoperatively without the need for reconstruction.

Reconstruction of the pelvis

General considerations

Adequate reconstruction is the key to a good functional outcome following pelvic resection. A number of options are available to reconstruct defects of the pelvis. In general, reconstructive options may be characterized as "prosthetic" (eg, hip arthroplasty, saddle prosthesis), "biologic" (eg, arthrodesis, the

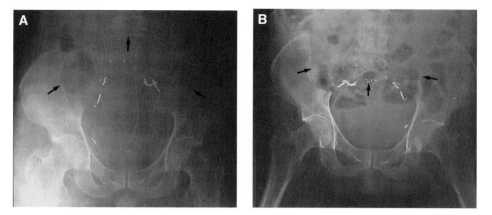

Fig. 5. Patient who underwent complete sacrectomy. Note the substantial translation of the lumbar spine as the patient goes from supine position (*A*) to sitting position (*B*).

use of allograft/autograft, pseudoarthrosis), or "combination," such as the allograft-prosthetic composite. Selection of the appropriate technique is a complex process that depends on a number of factors.

One should closely scrutinize the patient's medical history when deciding among reconstructive options. Any history of previous or current infection should be elicited, because the presence of persistent infection would preclude the use of prostheses or allograft materials. Those who are smokers or diabetics are also generally at higher risk for infection. Patients with frequent urinary tract infections should be evaluated and treated before reconstruction, especially when implantation of hardware or allograft is being considered [3,4]. Careful attention should be paid to whether the patient has received or will receive radiation therapy. Depending on the dose delivered, radiation can greatly diminish the body's ability to incorporate prostheses or heal grafts in the postreconstructive setting. The anticipated use of long-term steroids or other chemotherapeutic immunosuppressives should also be carefully considered, because they may have a propensity to hamper biologic incorporation of graft or prosthesis or to increase the risk for infection. One should also have an estimate of the longevity of the patient. In cases of metastatic disease, longevity may be limited, and therefore reconstructions should be performed in such a way as to limit perioperative morbidity and allow for early weight bearing and return to function.

The functional demands of the patient are important to consider when choosing a reconstruction technique. Younger patients are often more active and will almost certainly place more significant stresses on their reconstructions than will lower-demand patients (ie, thin, elderly). In addition to overall higher level of activity, the younger patient will require greater longevity from the reconstruction, assuming long-term survival. For these reasons, a durable and functional construct should be considered for this population. Fortunately, these patients also tend to have enhanced ability to accommodate biologic solutions. Patient habitus is another factor that may place demand on the reconstruction. In general, the higher the functional demand on the patient, the more one should lean toward the biologic reconstructions, whereas lower-demand patients (elderly, thin) may do better with prosthetic-type reconstructions.

The anticipated postoperative neurologic function is also important to consider in choosing a reconstruction technique. Because of the volumetric loss of the resected pelvis and the loss of any neurologic structures (and subsequently muscle tone) that may have been involved in the resection, soft tissue tensioning and balancing may be difficult to achieve. Any prosthetic reconstruction techniques that rely on soft tissue tensioning should therefore be approached with caution in this setting, because instability may be problematic. The implant system selected should provide the option of a constrained acetabular liner in the event that the surgeon believes that soft tissue compromise places the patient at high risk for dislocation.

The social situation of the patient should also be considered. Prosthetic-type reconstructions generally require adequate long-term follow-up, with frequent clinical and radiographic surveillance. If a patient's social situation is such that he or she is likely to be lost to follow-up, a more "permanent," durable, biologic type of reconstruction may be advisable.

One should also carefully consider the potential need for soft tissue coverage following reconstruction. With large pelvic or sacral resections, sizable soft tissue and bone defects often remain. With the introduction of avascular bone or metallic implants, the environment favors the development of infections, which can be devastating in these cases. In addition, the disruption of normal fascial planes around the abdomen and pelvis may result in painful or dangerous visceral herniations. Frequently, synthetic mesh is used to help close large defects. Any large pelvic or sacral resection should be undertaken with this in mind, and plastic surgery consultation should be considered.

Reconstruction of type I resections

Complete type I, I-S, or I-A resections generally require bony reconstruction to reconstitute mechanical continuity of the sacrum and acetabulum. This reconstruction is necessary to enable transmission of force from the lower extremity to the axial skeleton. The hip joint is not involved in these types of resections, and therefore prosthetic reconstructions are typically not indicated.

If the distance between the remaining ilium and the sacrum is small, a direct appositional iliosacral

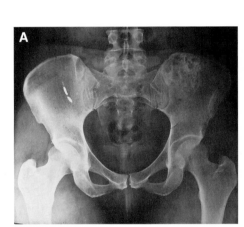

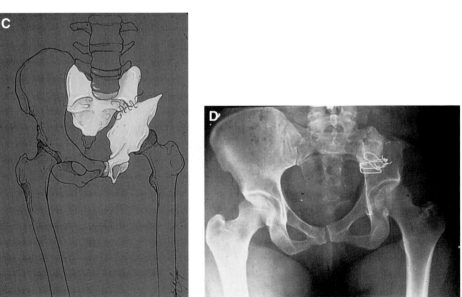

Fig. 6. (*A*) Anteroposterior pelvis radiograph shows chondrosarcoma of the left iliac wing. (*B*) With the iliac wing partially resected, the ilium is "closed down" and wired to the sacrum medially. (*C*) Diagram illustrating the procedure. (*D*) Postoperative radiograph.

arthrodesis may be performed (Fig. 6). The remaining sacroiliac joint is denuded of cartilage, and a wire or suture construct may be used to "close down" the pelvis by hinging the remaining hemipelvis through the flexible symphysis pubis joint anteriorly. Although this reconstruction alters hip joint mechanics somewhat, it does provide a durable sacroiliac arthrodesis, which heals readily owing to the compression of the two broad, flat, cancellous surfaces. The course of the sciatic nerve must be respected when performing this type of reconstruction. Occasionally, the inferior portion of the remaining ilium (sciatic notch) must be shaped to allow for egress of the sciatic nerve from the pelvis without mechanical impingement. The lower extremity should be immobilized in a spica cast postoperatively for 2 to 3 months, until clinical and radiographic bony union is achieved.

When the gap is too large to be closed using the direct apposition, a strut graft may be introduced to span the gap. Autograft fibular struts should be considered (with or without vascularity) in the setting of unfavorable biologic conditions (eg, smoking, diabetes,

infection, postradiation tissue, or anticipated radiation) to facilitate the bony healing. In younger patients with a favorable soft tissue envelope, allograft fibula is a good option that has been shown to incorporate reliably and avoids donor site morbidity (Fig. 7) [5]. Autoclaved autograft and vascularized iliac wing autograft have also been described in this setting.

Reconstruction of type II resections

These resections present the greatest challenges to reconstruction, because of the loss of the hip joint itself. A multitude of reconstructive options exist, and the principles described previously regarding the type of reconstruction to select should be considered.

Iliofemoral arthrodesis is an effective and durable means of reconstruction following resection of the acetabulum. This reconstruction may be achieved using many different techniques. The femoral head is osteotomized to produce a flat, cancellous surface, which is amenable to arthrodesis. The osteotomy on

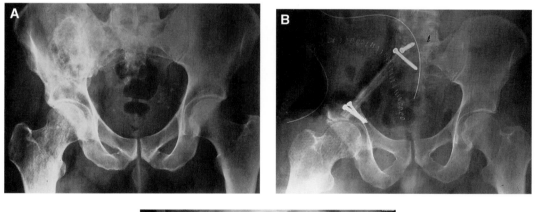

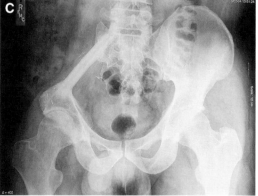

Fig. 7. (*A*) A type I resection is performed, resulting in pelvic discontinuity. (*B*) The defect is then reconstructed with a vascularized allograft. (*C*) Anteroposterior radiograph from 1 year postoperative shows solid incorporation.

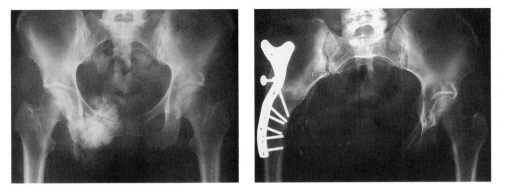

Fig. 8. Pre- and postoperative anteroposterior pelvis radiographs following resection of an osteogenic sarcoma and reconstruction by iliofemoral arthrodesis with "cobra" plate.

the femoral side should be made at or below the level of the base of the femoral neck, in the region where the blood supply is more robust and the likelihood of successful arthrodesis is increased. The superior femur may be "notched" to articulate with the iliac osteotomy. The femur is then apposed to the transverse resection along the iliac wing, using a "cobra"-type plate to achieve stability and compression (Fig. 8). Wiring techniques of fixation have also been described but are less stable. The patient must be protected postoperatively in a spica cast for 3 to 4 months to allow bony union to take place. Intercalary femoral allografts are occasionally used to minimize the postoperative limb-length discrepancy, but at the added cost of higher risk for nonunion and infection [6,7]. Extremity positioning is critical. The position of the lower extremity should be the same as that described for hip arthrodesis (0° adduction, 0° to

5° flexion, 5° external rotation) to maximize postoperative functionality. Once arthrodesis has been achieved, the patient is left with an extremely durable and functional reconstruction [8].

Ischiofemoral arthrodesis is another reconstructive option. This technique involves compressive fixation of the proximal femur to the adjacent ischium (Fig. 9). It has the advantage of maintaining more extremity length than is typically the case with an iliofemoral arthrodesis. This is a good option in those lacking sufficient ilium postresection to form an iliofemoral arthrodesis. Unfortunately, this construct is intrinsically less stable than that of an iliofemoral arthrodesis. Because of the presence of greater shear forces across the arthrodesis site, fusion is more difficult to achieve. In the Mayo experience, only about one third of these patients successfully progress to sound bony fusion. In addition, when solid is-

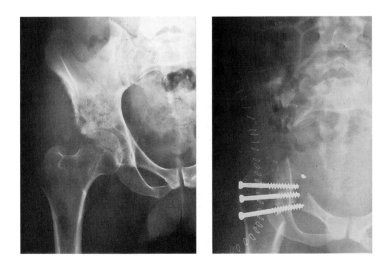

Fig. 9. Pre- and postoperative radiographs showing ischiofemoral arthrodesis after resection of a chondrosarcoma of the periacetabular region.

chiofemoral fusion is achieved, there is significant motion through the symphysis pubis, which may be painful for patients [9]. Because this construct is less stable, postoperative immobilization in a spica cast should last 3 to 4 months, followed by brace immobilization for another month or two until bony union is achieved.

Another option in the reconstruction of type II deficits is that of arthroplasty, in the form of allograft-prosthetic composite. The resected bone defect may be reconstituted, using either size-matched allograft pelvis or autoclaved autograft (if appropriate), which is fixed with the use of screws and plates (Fig. 10). These reconstructions function best when there is adequate host ischium and ilium remaining to support the construct and provide fixation. Once the bone is reconstituted, arthroplasty is performed using standard techniques. Constrained liners are often necessary to achieve hip stability, because the large soft tissue and regional neurologic insult results in little intrinsic

opportunity to stabilize the hip. The acetabular component should be redundantly stabilized in anticipation of high bone interface forces, because of the nature of the constrained liner and the incapacity of the host allograft (or autoclaved autograft) to ingrow effectively. Outcomes of this reconstruction are variable, with infection and stress fracture being commonly reported complications [10–12].

Following acetabular resection, reconstruction may also be performed with a "saddle" prosthesis (Fig. 11). This technique provides some stability for ambulation and maintains leg length of the patient. The prosthesis rests within a notch in the remaining ilium, which gives the construct vertical stability. The notch created for the prosthesis should be medialized, if possible, to reduce the torque on the remaining ilium. Eventually, the "articulating" portion of the prosthesis becomes encased in bony and fibrous tissues, which confer some degree of stability. Sutures passed through the prosthesis and into the ilium at the

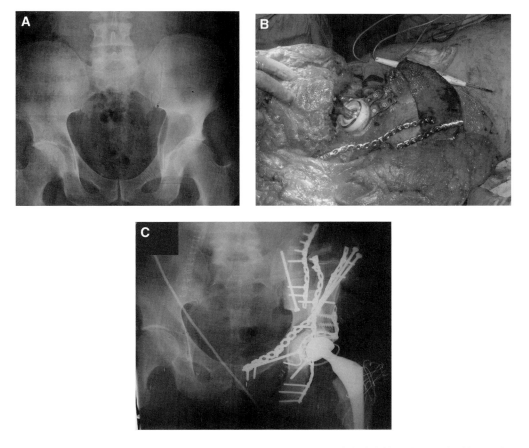

Fig. 10. Anteroposterior radiograph shows lesion in the periacetabular region of the left hip (*A*), treated with resection and reconstruction with allograft-prosthetic composite (*B*). (*C*) Postoperative radiograph.

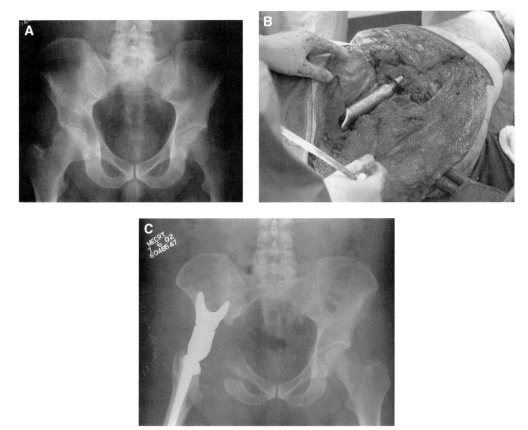

Fig. 11. A left periacetabular lesion (*A*) treated with resection and reconstruction using the "saddle" prosthesis (*B*). (*C*) Postoperative radiograph.

time of surgery may improve perioperative stability until the prosthesis is stabilized more lastingly by bone or scar formation. Proximal migration of these components over time has been reported, and instability can be an issue as well. Functional abductors facilitate this form of reconstruction, because they enhance the soft tissue tensioning necessary for stability [13].

At times, it is appropriate to leave patients with a pseudoarthrosis (Fig. 12). This guideline holds especially true for patients with deep-seated infections in which the introduction of prosthetic components or devascularized bone is not advisable. Pseudoarthroses do not involve the implantation of avascular bone or metallic prosthesis and therefore do not carry any of the associated morbidities. Although pseudoarthroses are not typically as functional as successful arthrodeses or prosthetic reconstructions, they can create a pain-free and moderately functional extremity [6,8].

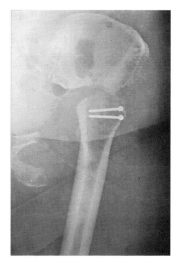

Fig. 12. Postoperative radiograph after type II pelvic resection and iliofemoral pseudoarthrosis.

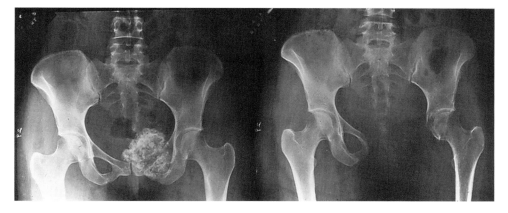

Fig. 13. Pre- and postoperative radiographs following type III pelvic resection. Note that the acetabulum remains in continuity with the axial skeleton.

Reconstruction of type III resections

Type III resections do not generally require skeletal reconstruction when acetabular stability can be maintained (Fig. 13). Patients are cautioned about postoperative loss of adduction strength and the potential for stress fractures and reactive changes in the iliosacral region. Function in these cases is typically good. Following these resections, patients have a propensity to form visceral or bladder hernias because of the defect created. Careful closure, which includes the use of sheet graft material or local tissue flaps (eg, vertical rectus flaps), should be considered.

Sacral reconstructions

Sagittal hemisacrectomies should be reconstructed by recreating bony continuity between the ilium and the remaining sacrum using auto- or allograft strut fixation. The technique is similar to that described earlier for strut reconstruction of type I pelvic resections. Again, autograft or vascularized struts should be considered in the patient population with anticipated healing difficulty (ie, smokers, diabetics, and patients who have tissue beds that have been previously radiated or those in whom postoperative radiation is anticipated).

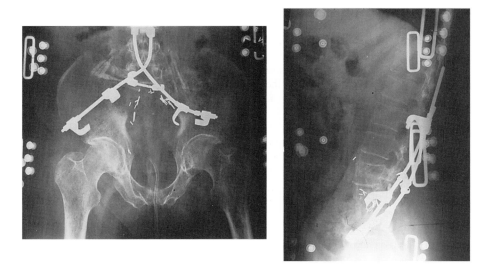

Fig. 14. This radiograph shows iliolumbar arthrodesis using techniques from the 1980s following sacral resection.

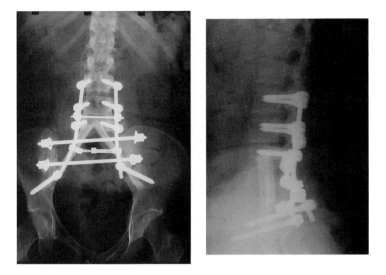

Fig. 15. This radiograph shows a "modern" reconstruction (iliolumbar arthrodesis) after total sacrectomy. Note the fibular struts in the triangular arrangement and the use of top-loaded screw and bar constructs.

Transverse hemisacrectomies involving most of the sacral ala and complete sacrectomies should be reconstructed using techniques of lumbo-iliac fusion. This procedure has been accomplished in the past with Luque- or Galvaston-type or rod and wire/hook constructs (Fig. 14). Current techniques use the newer generation of top-loaded rod and screw constructs for spinal fixation. Free or rotational (vertical rectus abdominis) flap coverage should be strongly considered after major resections of the sacrum, especially when devitalized bone (graft) material or hardware is to be implanted.

In performing this reconstruction, bilateral pedicle screws are placed at the L4 and L5 levels posteriorly.

An oval receptacle is created using a burr in the inferior endplate of the L5 vertebral body and anteriorly along the midaspect of the iliopectineal lines bilaterally. Four spinal fixation screws (two on each side) are also placed in an inside-out orientation within the ilium to provide the distal fixation. Two fibular grafts (auto- or allograft) are then placed distally within the previously created iliopectineal receptacles and proximally within the L5 receptacle to create a triangular construct. The fixation bars are bent and positioned, and laminar spreaders are used to compress the construct. The bars are then tightly secured. Bone graft is placed at the distal and proximal receptacles, as well as in the posterolateral aspects of the L4 and L5 transverse processes to facilitate solid bony arthrodesis (Figs. 15 and 16).

Summary

Partial resections of the pelvis and sacrum are complex procedures. Depending on the location and extent of the resection, patients may experience significant postoperative morbidity. The bony and soft tissue reconstructions should be approached with careful forethought. A thorough knowledge of the reconstructive options with their respective indications is essential to engagement in this type of surgery. The initial focus should be on adequate resection of the lesion, followed by restoration or maintenance of stability.

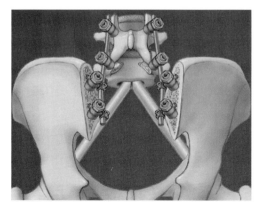

Fig. 16. The "modern" iliolumbar arthrodesis technique.

References

[1] Enneking WF, Dunham WK. Resection and reconstruction for primary neoplasms involving the innominate bone. J Bone Joint Surg 1978;60A(6):731–46.

[2] Gunterberg B, Romanus B, Stener B. Pelvic strength after major amputation of the sacrum. An experimental study. Acta Orthop Scand 1976;47:635–42.

[3] Hillmann A, Hoffmann C, Gosheger G, et al. Tumors of the pelvis: complications after reconstruction. Arch Orthop Trauma Surg 2003;123(7):340–4.

[4] Haley RW, Culver DH, Morgan WM, et al. Identifying patients at high risk of surgical wound infection. A simple multivariate index of patient susceptibility and wound contamination. Am J Epidemiol 1985;121:206–15.

[5] Cannon SR, Tillman RM, Grimer RJ, et al. Treatment of primary bone tumors of the ilium by local resection and fibular strut graft (non-vascularized) [abstract]. In: Companacci M, Capanna R, editors. Proceedings of the Eighth International Symposium on Limb Salvage. May 10–12, 1995, Vol. 77. Florence (Italy): International Symposium on Limb Salvage; 1995.

[6] O'Connor M. Malignant pelvic tumors: limb sparing resection and reconstruction. Semin Surg Oncol 1997;13:49–54.

[7] Capanna R, Donati D, Fazioli F, et al. Iliofemoral arthrodesis with intercalary allograft. In: Brown KL, editor. Complications of limb salvage: proceedings of the Sixth International Symposium on Limb Salvage. September 8–11, 1991. Montreal (Canada): International Symposium on Limb Salvage; 1991. p. 205–9.

[8] Fuchs B, O'Connor MI, Kaufman KR, et al. Iliofemoral arthrodesis and pseudoarthrosis: a long-term functional outcome evaluation. Clin Orthop 2002;397:29–35.

[9] Tomeno B, Languepin A, Gerber C. Local resection with limb salvage for the treatment of periacetabular bone tumors: functional results in nine cases. In: Enneking WF, editor. Limb salvage and musculoskeletal oncology. New York: Churchill Livingstone; 1987. p. 147–56.

[10] Donati D, Capanna R, Caldora P, et al. Internal hemipelvectomy of the acetabular area using different methods of reconstruction. In: Tan SK, editor. Limb salvage: current trends. Proceedings of the Seventh International Symposium on Limb Salvage. August 23–7, 1993. Singapore: International Symposium on Limb Salvage; 1993. p. 185–8.

[11] Harrington KD. The use of hemipelvic allografts or autoclaved grafts for reconstruction after wide resections of malignant tumors of the pelvis. J Bone Joint Surg 1992;74A:331–41.

[12] Rosenberg AG, Mankin HJ. Complications of allograft surgery. In: Epps Jr CH, editor. Complications in orthopedic surgery, Vol. 2. 2nd edition. Philadelphia: JB Lippincott; 1986. p. 1385–417.

[13] Neider E, Friesecke C. Mid-term results of 73 saddle prostheses, endo model, at total hip revision arthroplasty [abstract]. In: Tan SK, editor. Limb salvage: current trends. Proceedings of the Seventh International Symposium on Limb Salvage. August 23–7, 1993. Singapore: International Symposium on Limb Salvage; 1993. p. 313.

ELSEVIER
SAUNDERS

Orthop Clin N Am 37 (2006) 99–104

ORTHOPEDIC
CLINICS
OF NORTH AMERICA

Surgical Management of Metastatic Spine Tumors

Safdar N. Khan, MD*, Rakesh Donthineni, MD

*Department of Orthopaedic Surgery, University of California at Davis Medical Center, 4860 Y Street, Suite 3800,
Sacramento, CA 95817, USA*

Recent advances in diagnostic tests and radiologic imaging, and the development of novel chemotherapeutic agents and radiation methods have greatly altered the treatment options in patients who have spinal tumors. Improvements in fundamental understanding of the mechanisms of bone metastases, developments in spinal instrumentation, and recent introduction of recombinant bone morphogenetic proteins for spinal reconstruction offer promising strategies in selected patients [1]. Clear applications of the fundamental surgical oncology still apply to spinal tumors. This article considers recent advances in management of the metastatic tumors to the spine.

Several factors have led to the dramatic changes in the approach to metastasis to the spine. Improvements in surgical approaches to the entire vertebral column have made it feasible to resect tumors involving spine at nearly all levels. Development of third and fourth generation instrumentation allows the spine surgeon to reconstruct vertebral segments infiltrated with tumor. Improvement in radiologic diagnosis of tumors caused by the widespread use of MRI, CT, and positron emission tomography (PET) scanning has enhanced the ability to visualize the specific tumors and their extensions. This visualization allows adequate surgical approach and postoperative assessment of therapy. Recent advances in chemotherapeutics offer promise for treatment that was not feasible even a few years ago [2–4].

Despite these understandings, the surgical treatment of metastatic spinal tumors is not standardized. Most clinical studies remain retrospective reviews spanning several decades, with inconsistent treatment modalities.

Certain staging systems have been used to divide spinal tumors. The Enneking staging system divides benign tumors into three stages [1–3] and localized malignant tumors into low or high grade (I or II) and intra- or extracompartmental (A or B). Metastatic sarcomas are staged as III, and often further classified as IIIA or IIIB, depending on if the primary tumor is intra- or extracompartmental. This classification is based on a complete initial evaluation that includes clinical features as discovered on history and physical examination, radiographic patterns, CT scans, and MRI data. Metastatic status can be determined with chest CT scans and a whole body bone scan. PET scans have been shown to be of value for sarcomas, although not fully used in all the treating centers. A tissue biopsy is needed to confirm the diagnosis and help plan the treatment.

To better understand the surgical approach and operative management of spinal tumors, it is important to review specific terminology. Curettage and intralesional describe the piecemeal removal of tumors from within the lesion, leaving gross tumor behind. Marginal resection is when the dissection is along the reactive zone (pseudocapsule) and may leave microscopic foci of the malignant tumor behind. Wide resection occurs when the dissection leaves a cuff of normal tissue around the tumor while allowing removal of the microscopic tumor foci. Radical resection refers to the removal of the whole compartment (ie, the whole affected bone) or individual muscle compartment.

---

* Corresponding author.
E-mail address: safdar.khan@ucdmc.ucdavis.edu
(S.N. Khan).

Epidemiology

The American Cancer Society estimates that approximately 2000 new cases of primary bone cancers and 6000 cases of soft tissue sarcomas are diagnosed in the United States each year [5]. Approximately 5% of these cases involve the spine. The incidence of primary spinal neoplasms is estimated to be 2.5 to 8.5 per 100,000 people per year [6]. Some bone tumors have a special predilection for the vertebral column. As a general rule, two important clinical features need to be considered in evaluating the potential malignancy of the lesion in the spine: age and location. More than 75% of lesions located in the vertebral body are malignant, whereas only one third of lesions in the posterior elements are malignant. Secondly, more than two thirds of all lesions seen in the pediatric population under 18 years of age are benign, whereas greater than two thirds of all lesions are malignant in adults.

Metastasis to the spine is a common feature of many solid tumors. Approximately 1.3 million new cases of cancer are diagnosed annually in the United States, of which 40% to 50% will die of uncontrolled metastatic disease [7]. Autopsy studies have revealed that between 5% and 30% of all cancer patients have had metastasis to the spine, of which 20% are clinically symptomatic. In most retrospective reviews, four primary sites alone can account for more than two thirds of all metastasis to the spine, breast, lung, hematopoietic/lymphoid system, and prostate.

Evaluation of metastatic tumors

The axial skeleton is the third most common site of metastases from systemic cancer. It has been estimated that nearly 10% of patients who have spinal metastasis become symptomatic with pathologic fractures requiring surgical intervention. Metastasis to the spine from systemic tumors can result from several mechanisms, including hematogenous spread, local extension through lymphatics, and extension through intervertebral foramen. The literature has defined four common primary sites that predominate for metastasis to the spine: breast, prostate, lung, and the hematopoietic system.

The use of bisphosphonates is among the recent advances for the reduction of morbidity in skeletal fractures and pain from spinal metastasis. Second-generation bisphosphonates such as pamidronate and zoledronate have been used with considerable success.

History

The most common presenting complaint in patients presenting with spinal metastasis is pain. The characteristics of pain are often described as unrelenting, nonmechanical, and progressive. Although the pain is primarily axial early in the disease process, neural compression may lead to radiculopathy. Neurologic symptoms appear to be the primary reason patients present to spinal surgeons. Gilbert and colleagues [8] revealed that motor weakness was a presenting symptom in 76% of patients, including 17% of patients who were paralyzed at presentation. Paresthesias were reported in nearly 50% of patients. Other items to focus on when taking patient history include initial presentation of neurologic deficit, progressive nature of the deficit, weight loss, anorexia, fatigue, tobacco use, and family history of malignancy.

Physical examination

Physical examination in these patients must include a thorough examination of areas that may be affected by most primary tumors, including the breasts, chest, abdomen, prostate, and lymphatic system. Neurologic exam must be as detailed as possible and painstakingly documented for future reference. Localized spinal tenderness may represent underlying tumor. Radicular pain and sensorimotor examination often accurately localize the tumor to within one of two vertebral levels.

Radiographs

Patients who have metastatic spine tumors are evaluated primarily because of pain or new neurologic deficits. To determine the extent of systemic disease, accurate assessment of the spinal segments involved, including staging studies, need to be performed. The workup includes plain radiographs; radiographic and radionucleotide imaging; CT scanning; and MRI and PET scans.

The major advantages of CT scans are its wide availability and low cost in comparison to MRIs. Image manipulation using appropriate window width and levels must be performed. CT scans are now more reliable in demonstrating cortical outlines and calcifications in comparison to MRIs. CT also allows proper needle placement when needle biopsies are indicated. Currently, CT-guided systems are also used for intraoperative navigation and correct placements of pedicle screws.

MRI has largely revolutionized the evaluation of spinal tumors. This imaging allows tumor assessment in multiplanar dimensions and assessment of the entire spine, and detects early marrow invasion in multifocal involvement with great precision.

Indications for surgical management

Indications for surgical reconstruction of symptomatic metastasis remain controversial. Data from nonrandomized trials suggest that patients who have impaired motor function may benefit equally from surgery as from radiation therapy. However, recent work by Sundaresan and colleagues [9] suggests that direct anterior ablation with surgical stabilization provides superior ambulatory rates and pain relief than historically used posterior laminectomy. Several factors have strengthened arguments for the role of primary surgery in the treatment of spinal metastasis. These factors include decreasing mortality rates of surgery with improvements in neurologic outcome and duration of palliation. Improvements in spinal instrumentation, particularly the use of pedicle screw instrumentation, have greatly reduced the morbidity of posterior instrumentation. Pedicle screw fixation allows superior stabilization, shorter segment fixation, and more effective three-column fixation. Currently, the indications for operative intervention include progressive neurologic deficit before, during, and after radiation therapy; intractable pain unresponsive to conservative therapy; need for histologic diagnosis; radioresistant tumors; and spinal instability or vertebral collapse with or without neurologic compromise.

The goals of reconstructive spinal surgery include minimizing morbidity, neural decompression, tumor debulking and resection, and anterior–posterior stabilization. In general, the posterior procedure for stabilization is performed first with pedicle screws. The posterior elements are removed and the pedicles resected to allow access to the vertebral body. This approach obviates the need for extensive transcavitary approaches. Patients who have life expectancies greater than 1 year may benefit from a second-staged anterior procedure to provide anterior column support. The anterior column may be reconstructed with titanium mesh cages filled with autogenous bone graft or recombinant growth factors.

Prognostic factors

Tomita and colleagues [10] designed a new surgical strategy for treatment of patients who have spinal metastases. These investigators reviewed 67 patients who had spinal metastases and had been treated from 1987 to 1991, and evaluated prognostic factors retrospectively (phase 1). A new scoring system for spinal metastases that was designed based on these data consists of three prognostic factors: (1) grade of malignancy (slow growth: one point; moderate growth: two points; rapid growth: four points), (2) visceral metastases (no metastasis: zero points; treatable: two points: untreatable: four points), and (3) bone metastases (solitary or isolated: one point; multiple: two points). These three factors were added together to give a prognostic score between 2 and 10. The treatment goal for each patient was set according to this prognostic score. The strategy for each patient was decided along with the treatment goal: a prognostic score of 2 to 3 points suggested a wide or marginal excision for long-term local control; 4 to 5 points indicated marginal or intralesional excision for middle-term local control; 6 to 7 points justified palliative surgery for short-term palliation; and 8 to 10 points indicated nonoperative supportive care. According to this surgical strategy, 61 patients were treated prospectively between 1993 and 1996 (phase 2). The extent of the spinal metastases was stratified using the surgical classification of spinal tumors, and technically appropriate and feasible surgery was performed, such as en bloc spondylectomy, piecemeal thorough excision, curettage, or palliative surgery. The mean survival time of the 28 patients treated with wide or marginal excision was 38.2 months (26 had successful local control). The mean survival time of the 13 patients treated with intralesional excision was 21.5 months (9 had successful local control). The mean survival time of the 11 patients treated with palliative surgery and stabilization was 10.1 months (8 had successful local control). The mean survival time of the patients who had terminal care was 5.3 months. This strategy provided appropriate guidelines for treatment in all patients who had spinal metastases.

Surgical approach and outcome

In recent years it has been recognized that the surgical treatment of spinal metastatic disease requires more than just removal of the tumor. Most spinal tumors originate in the vertebral body with spinal cord compression anteriorly. Factors contributing to the anterior compression include vertebral body collapse, fracture, or kyphotic angulation. Several studies have examined the role of vertebrectomies, vertebral body reconstruction, and fusion;

however, not all patients are candidates for such aggressive intervention.

Among a series of 740 spinal tumors treated in Hannover, Germany, Klekamp and Samii [11] operated on 106 spinal metastases in 101 patients. Of the tumors that were operated on by Klekamp, 79% were operated on using a posterolateral approach, 12% using an anterior approach, and the remaining 9% using an anterior and posterior approach. Complete resection was achieved for 43.4% of the metastases, whereas 48.1% were removed partially and 7.5% were biopsied. Surgery was followed by radiotherapy, chemotherapy, or hormone treatment, based on the type of tumor. The overall local recurrence rates as determined by the Kaplan Meier method were 57.9% after 6 months, 69.3% after 1 year, and 96% after 4 years. Multiple regression analyses revealed that significant, independent predictors of a low rate of local metastatic recurrence included preoperative status of ambulation, favorable tumor histology, cervical level, complete resection, low number of affected vertebral bodies, and elective surgery. Postoperative neurologic outcome was related to preoperative neurologic deficits. Of the patients walking preoperatively, 96% were able to do so at least 3 months postoperatively. However, only 22% of patients unable to walk regained walking capacity for 3 months. Among the patient population operated on by Klekamp, 89% remained continent of urine postoperatively for 3 months, whereas only 31% regained sphincter control for this amount of time postoperatively. Longer survival times were demonstrated for patients who had favorable tumor histology, independent ambulation, long history, male gender, cervical level, complete resection, posterior approach, no additional metastases in other organs, and no instability. The overall survival rates were 58.8% after 6 months, 48% after 1 year, and 19.5% after 5 years postoperatively. The study by Klekamp and Samii concluded that reconstructive surgery had a place in the treatment of patients who had metastatic disease of the spine with concurrently presenting neurologic symptoms or spinal instability.

A subpopulation of patients who have spinal metastases often has patterns of disease requiring an anterior and posterior surgical decompression and spinal fusion. For patients whose debilitating illness or prior surgery makes an anterior approach challenging, a posterior transpedicular approach may be used to resect the involved vertebral bodies, posterior elements, and epidural tumor. Bilsky and colleagues [12] assessed neurologic and functional outcome of patients who had metastatic spinal cord compression using a posterolateral transpedicular ap-

proach with circumferential fusion. In their series, 25 patients were operated on using a posterolateral transpedicular approach. The primary indications for surgery included back pain (15 patients) and neurologic progression (10 patients). All patients had vertebral body disease, and 21 patients had high-grade spinal cord compression from epidural disease as assessed by MRI. In each patient, the anterior column was reconstructed with polymethyl methacrylate and Steinmann pins and the posterior column with long segmental pedicle screw fixation. In their patients, neurologic symptoms were stable or improved in 23 patients. In the remaining 2 patients, 1 patient who had an acute myelopathy was immediately worse after surgery, and 1 patient had a delayed neurologic worsening that eventually progressed to paraplegia. The investigators concluded that a posterolateral transpedicular approach provided a wide surgical exposure to decompress and instrument the anterior and posterior spine. They recommended this technique as it avoided the morbidity associated with anterior approaches and provided immediate stability.

Anterior-alone surgery for the treatment of spinal tumors has gained acceptance; however, Gokaslan and colleagues [13] reviewed their results in patients who underwent anterior vertebral body resection, reconstruction, and stabilization for spinal metastases limited to the thoracic region. They reviewed 72 patients who had metastatic spinal tumors treated by transthoracic vertebrectomy. The primary tumors included renal cancer in 19 patients, breast cancer in 10, melanoma or sarcoma in 10, and lung cancer in 9. The most common presenting symptoms were back pain, which occurred in 90% of patients, and lower-extremity weakness, which occurred in 64% of patients. All patients underwent transthoracic vertebrectomy, decompression, reconstruction with methylmethacrylate, and anterior fixation with locking plate and screw constructs. Supplemental posterior instrumentation was required in seven patients who had disease involving the cervicothoracic or thoracolumbar junction, which was causing severe kyphosis. Their results indicated that with this approach, pain improved in 60 of 65 patients. This improvement was found to be statistically significant ($P < .001$) based on visual analog scales and narcotic analgesic medication use. Of the 46 patients, 35 who presented with neurologic dysfunction improved significantly ($P < .001$) following the procedure. The one-year survival rate for the entire study population was 62%.

Gokaslan and colleagues' [13] results indicated that transthoracic vertebrectomy and spinal stabilization could benefit select patients presenting with spinal metastasis by restoring or preserving ambulation and by controlling intractable spinal pain.

The treatment of metastatic lesions in the thoracic spine has received a lot of attention because 70% of cases involve this region. The lumbar spine is less frequently involved (20% cases), and it is unclear whether its unique anatomic and biomechanical features affect surgery-related outcomes. Holman and colleagues [14] reviewed a series of patients who had lumbar metastatic lesions, assessing neurologic and pain outcomes, complications, and survival. Data were reviewed in 139 patients who underwent 166 surgical procedures for lumbar metastatic disease. Pain was the most common presenting symptom (96%), including local pain, radicular pain, and axial pain caused by instability. Patients underwent anterior, posterior, and combined approaches depending on the anatomic distribution of disease or the presence of instability. Their results showed that 94% of the cases demonstrated complete or partial improvement in pain up to 1 month after surgery. These data indicated that the surgical treatment of metastatic lesions in the lumbar spine improved neurologic and ambulatory function and significantly reduced axial spinal pain, and that results were comparable with those for other spinal regions. The investigators indicated, however, that when lumbar vertebrectomy was required, anterior approaches minimized blood loss and wound-related complications.

Surgical resection for solitary lesions

Sundaresan and colleagues [15] analyzed the long-term survival, neurologic outcome, and results of surgery in a well-defined subset of patients who had solitary spinal lesions attributed to metastatic primaries. A retrospective review of 80 consecutive patients who had solitary sites of spine involvement from solid tumors analyzed several outcome measures, including clinical parameters, neurologic grade, preoperative pain, and radiologic evaluation. This review evaluated survival analysis and prognostic factors for long-term survival. The overall median survival after surgery was 30 months, with 18% surviving 5 years or more. Most importantly, however, survival varied by tumor type, with the best prognosis noted in patients who had breast or kidney cancer. The surgical morbidity was significantly higher in those receiving prior irradiation, and the local recurrence rate also increased in patients who had received prior irradiation.

Risk factors and incidence of complications

Wise and colleagues [16] examined the risk factors for complications, incidence of complications, and survival rates in patients who had metastatic disease of the spine. They reviewed 80 patients undergoing surgical treatment for metastatic disease of the spine. Surgical indications included progressive neurologic deficit; neurologic deficit failing to respond to or progressing after radiation treatment; intractable pain; radioresistant tumors; or the need for histologic diagnosis. Patients underwent anterior, posterior, or combined decompression and stabilization procedures. In their series, 65 patients showed no change in Frankel grade, 19 improved one Frankel grade, and 1 deteriorated one Frankel grade, and 1 patient had paraplegia. Thirty-five complications occurred in 20 patients (25.0%); 10 patients (12.5%) had multiple complications accounting for 23 of the 35 postoperative problems (65.7%); and 60 patients had no surgical complications (75%). The investigators' data suggested that the likelihood of a complication occurring was related to Harrington classifications (I: no neurologic involvement or minor sensory impairment; II: bony involvement without collapse or instability; III: major neurologic impairment (sensory of motor) without significant bony involvement; IV: vertebral collapse with mechanical pain or instability but without significant neurologic compromise; V: vertebral collapse/instability combined with major neurologic impairment), demonstrating significant neurologic deficits and the use of preoperative radiation therapy. In general, Harrington classifications with neurologic deficits and lower Frankel grades before and after surgery were associated with an increased risk for complication. The investigators concluded that to minimize complications, patients must be carefully selected based on expected length of survival, the use of radiation therapy, presence of neurologic deficit, and impending spinal instability or collapse caused by bone destruction.

Quality of life after surgery

Regardless of surgical approach and postoperative stability, satisfactory quality of life and high patient acceptance are essential in surgical reconstructive procedures. Weigel and colleagues [17] evaluated the postoperative outcome and quality of life of 76 patients surgically treated for symptomatic spinal metastases. The investigators treated patients who primarily had anterior decompression and fusion. Neurologic improvement with regard to Frankel classification was observed in 58% of the patients, and 93% were able to walk postoperatively. Pain relief was noted in 89%. Overall, 67% of the patients achieved moderate or good general health as shown by the Karnofsky Index, and 80% were satisfied or very satisfied with the surgical intervention. A testament to the high-risk nature of these patients, 19% of the surgical interventions were associated with complications, local tumor recurrence developed in 22% of the patients, and paraplegia ultimately developed in 18% of patients. The investigators concluded that anterior surgery was of benefit in most metastatic lesions in terms of satisfactory postoperative outcome and quality of life. However, in patients who had melanoma or lung carcinoma, the investigators advocated spinal intervention surgery only in very exceptional cases.

Reflections

The treatment of patients who have metastatic spine disease remains a challenging surgical problem. To optimize surgical efficacy and postoperative quality of life, it is essential that these patients be treated with a multidisciplinary effort. Treatment goals and indications for surgical management must be reviewed clearly with the patient. Adjuvant treatment such as radiation should be considered if clearly beneficial regarding tumor growth and obviating surgery, although it can be used in conjunction with surgery either pre- or postoperatively. Eligible patients must have a reasonable life expectancy, and a course of nonoperative therapy must have failed. Surgical approach must be made based on the location of epidural compression or instability.

References

[1] Khan SN, Lane JM. The use of recombinant human bone morphogenetic protein-2 (rhBMP-2) in orthopaedic applications. Expert Opin Biol Ther 2004;4(5): 741–8.

[2] Chiras J, Adem C, Vallee JN, et al. Selective intra-arterial chemoembolization of pelvic and spine bone metastases. Eur Radiol 2004;14(10):1774–80.

[3] Kato T, Sato K, Sasaki R, et al. Targeted cancer chemotherapy with arterial microcapsule chemoembolization: review of 1013 patients. Cancer Chemother Pharmacol 1996;37(4):289–96.

[4] Fiorentini G, Rossi S, Bonechi F, et al. Intra-arterial hepatic chemoembolization in liver metastases from neuroendocrine tumors: a phase II study. J Chemother 2004;16(3):293–7.

[5] Herzog CE. Overview of sarcomas in the adolescent and young adult population. J Pediatr Hematol Oncol 2005;27(4):215–8.

[6] Perrin RG, Laxton AW. Metastatic spine disease: epidemiology, pathophysiology, and evaluation of patients. Neurosurg Clin N Am Oct 2004;15(4):365–73.

[7] North RB, LaRocca VR, Schwartz J, et al. Surgical management of spinal metastases: analysis of prognostic factors during a 10-year experience. J Neurosurg Spine 2005;2(5):564–73.

[8] Gilbert RW, Kim JH, Posner JB, et al. Epidural spinal cord compression from metastatic tumor: diagnosis and treatment. Ann Neurol 1978;3(1):40–51.

[9] Sundaresan N, Boriani S, Rothman A, et al. Tumors of the osseous spine. J Neurooncol 2004;69(1–3): 273–90.

[10] Tomita K, Kawahara N, Kobayashi T, et al. Surgical strategy for spinal metastases. Spine 2001;26(3): 298–306.

[11] Klekamp J, Samii M. Surgical results for spinal meningiomas. Surg Neurol 1999;52(6):552–62.

[12] Bilsky MH, Boland P, Lis E, et al. Single-stage posterolateral transpedicle approach for spondylectomy, epidural decompression, and circumferential fusion of spinal metastases. Spine 2000;25(17):2240–9.

[13] Gokaslan ZL, York JE, Walsh GL, et al. Transthoracic vertebrectomy for metastatic spinal tumors. J Neurosurg 1998;89(4):599–609.

[14] Holman PJ, Suki D, McCutcheon I. Surgical management of metastatic disease of the lumbar spine: experience with 139 patients. J Neurosurg Spine 2005; 2(5):550–63.

[15] Sundaresan N, Rothman A, Manhart K, et al. Surgery for solitary metastases of the spine: Rationale and results of treatment. Spine 2002;27(16):1802–6.

[16] Wise JJ, Fischgrund JS, Herkowitz HN, et al. Complication, survival rates, and risk factors of surgery for metastatic disease of the spine. Spine 1999;24(18): 1943–51.

[17] Weigel B, Maghsudi M, Neumann C, et al. Surgical management of symptomatic spinal metastases. Postoperative outcome and quality of life. Spine 1999; 24(21):2240–6.

ELSEVIER
SAUNDERS

Orthop Clin N Am 37 (2006) 105–112

ORTHOPEDIC
CLINICS
OF NORTH AMERICA

Image-Guided Therapies in Orthopedic Oncology

Tarun Sabharwal, FRCSI, FRCR[a],*, Richard Salter, MRCS, FRCR[a],
Andreas Adam, FRCP, FRCS, FRCR[a], Afshin Gangi, MD, PhD[a,b]

[a]Department of Radiology, Guy's and St. Thomas' Hospital, Lambeth Palace Road, London, UK SE1 7EH
[b]Department of Radiology, University Louis Pasteur, University Hospital of Strasbourg,
1 Place de l'Hôpital, BP 426–67091, Strasbourg, France

Tumors of bone can present many management problems, and a thorough knowledge of the pathology, imaging, and treatment of these lesions is essential. In this article, the authors outline the minimally invasive techniques for the diagnosis and treatment of primary and secondary bone tumors.

Patients' symptoms and signs can be diverse (eg, pain, mechanical instability, or compression of vital structures). Surgery, often combined with adjuvant chemotherapy/radiotherapy, provides the only chance of cure. The remaining established treatments are primarily palliative and include radiotherapy, chemotherapy, hormonal treatment, radiopharmaceuticals, bisphosphonates, and analgesics. Despite this impressive range of treatment options, a number of patients are not suitable candidates or do not derive significant benefit (eg, patients who have localized bone pain secondary to metastatic tumor infiltration). External beam radiotherapy is the often the first treatment modality used for these patients [1,2]; however, 20% to 30% of treated patients do not experience pain relief [3]. These patients may benefit from novel percutaneous interventions that offer the advantages of being minimally invasive, effective, and repeatable.

The aim of this review is to outline percutaneous techniques that may be useful for the diagnosis and treatment of these patients. In particular, the existing procedures of percutaneous biopsy, alcoholization (ethanol ablation), vertebroplasty, kyphoplasty, osteoplasty, radiofrequency ablation, laser photocoagulation, and arterial embolization are reviewed. Aspects of each technique, including mechanism of action, patient selection, treatment technique, and recent patient outcome are presented.

Percutaneous needle biopsy

An open biopsy is considered by many to be the "gold standard" against which other biopsy methods should be judged. The large amount of tissue obtained gives the best chance of a representative sample being obtained. Despite this, many centers have moved toward percutaneous needle biopsy because of the advantages of low cost, improved patient comfort, and low rate of complications.

Percutaneous needle biopsy includes fine-needle aspiration and core-needle biopsy. The diagnoses of metastatic carcinoma and recurrent sarcoma are well suited to needle biopsy. Imaging is used to target the tumor and to identify areas of high diagnostic yield. Depending on the location, type of tumor, and operator experience, CT, ultrasound, or fluoroscopy can be used. These targeting techniques allow a diagnosis to be made in 85% to 90% of cases [4]. To optimize these methods, there should be close cooperation between the surgeon, pathologist, and radiologist involved.

Murphy and colleagues [5], in a large review of 9500 percutaneous skeletal biopsies, identified 22 complications (0.2%). They reported 9 pneumothoraces, 3 cases of meningitis, and 5 spinal cord injuries. Serious neurologic injury occurred in 0.08% of procedures. Death occurred in 0.02% of procedures.

* Corresponding author.
E-mail address: tarun.sabharwal@gstt.nhs.uk (T. Sabharwal).

It is likely that in the future, MRI-directed biopsies will become increasingly used. The superb tissue contrast offered by MRI in concert with MR spectrography to help target viable tumor will offer improved rates of diagnostic samples being obtained. Currently MRI can be used to place titanium marker coils. These coils are placed preoperatively, marking the periphery of the tumor. The coils are easily imaged with fluoroscopy intraoperatively, allowing complete surgical resection and reduced operating time [6].

Percutaneous ethanol ablation

Ethanol causes dehydration of the cytoplasm and subsequent coagulation necrosis followed by fibrous reaction. Within vessels, ethanol induces necrosis of endothelial cells and platelet aggregation, thus causing thrombosis and tissue ischemia. Percutaneous alcoholization of bone metastasis is indicated when patients have painful severe osteolytic bone metastases and conventional anticancer therapy is ineffective, when high doses of opiates are necessary to control pain, or when rapid pain relief is necessary (radiation or chemotherapy usually have a 2- to 4-week lag) (Figs. 1–3) [7,8].

One of the major advantages of the injection of alcohol into bone metastasis is the rapid relief of pain that occurs within 24 to 48 hours, with best results being obtained with small metastases (diameters ranging from 3–6 cm). Ethanol injection is painful, and alcohol instillation should be performed while

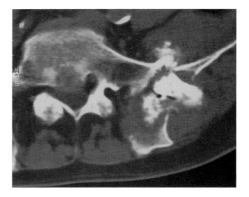

Fig. 2. Percutaneous alcohol injection. Following the injection of contrast and local anesthetic, ethanol is instilled.

using a combination of an opioid analgesia and a sedative agent to minimize the discomfort.

Pain relief has been reported as satisfactory in up to 74% of patients, with the duration of relief lasting from 10 to 27 weeks (9-month maximal survival in this group). Twenty-three percent of patients had recurrence of their pain after 2 to 4 months post treatment due to tumor progression [6].

The major contraindication to this technique is when there is risk of the alcohol diffusing into vital structures or intra-articularly [9]. A common side effect following this treatment is postembolization syndrome (fever and malaise in the first 72 hours). Other complications include neural injury and hyperuricemia following massive necrosis of tumor after injection of large volumes (>30 mL) of alcohol [6].

In addition to pain relief, mechanical stability is a consideration in weight-bearing regions. In this situation, ethanol injection may not be sufficient on its own and percutaneous osteoplasty should be considered.

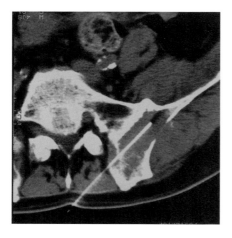

Fig. 1. Percutaneous alcohol injection. Percutaneous needle placement into a destructive metastasis of the ilium.

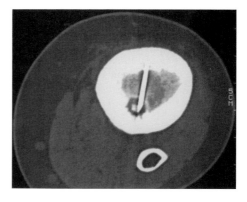

Fig. 3. Percutaneous laser ablation. Laser fiber placement in tibial osteoid osteoma.

Laser photocoagulation

The first interstitial thermal ablation of a tumor performed with laser therapy was reported in 1983. Since then, experimental studies have shown that a reproducible thermal injury can be produced with near–infrared wavelength lasers (Nd:YAG diode laser, 800–1000 nm wavelength). Nd:YAG lasers have been used to treat tumors of the esophagus, stomach, colon, and pulmonary bronchus. The first use of lasers to treat patients who had bone tumors was reported in 1993. Lasers are intense light sources that use light energy to produce their tissue effect. These properties enable reliable and direct transmission of high amounts of energy over long distances. Laser energy, with its powerful and precise ability to ablate, coagulate, and vaporize dense tissues and being transmissible in optical fiber, is an ideal tool for use in percutaneous ablations.

Interstitial laser photocoagulation consists of percutaneous insertion of optical fibers into the tumor. The tumor is coagulated and destroyed by direct heating. From a single, bare 400-mm laser fiber, light at optical or near–infrared wavelength scatters within tissue and is converted into heat. Light energy of 2.0 W produces a spherical volume of coagulative necrosis 1.6 cm in diameter in bone, whereas use of higher power results in charring and vaporization around the fiber tip. For producing larger volumes of necrosis (>1.6 cm), it is necessary to fire multiple bare fibers arrayed at 1.5- to 2-cm spacing throughout a target lesion. Portable solid-state diode lasers (Diomed, Cambridge, England) are now available with power outputs up to 60 W. This energy can be delivered through fibers over 10 m in length, with the great advantage of being fully compatible with MRI [10]. The indications and contraindications for laser ablation are the same as those for radiofrequency ablation. With a low-power laser technique, a very well defined coagulation volume of predictable size and shape can be obtained in bone tissue. The small size of the coagulation necrosis, however, limits its use in large tumors. The best indications are osteoid osteoma and contraindications of the other ablation techniques.

Osteoid osteoma is a benign neoplasm of bone and occurs more often in men. The age range is from 2 to 50 years, but 90% of these tumors occur before age 25 years. Osteoid osteoma produces local pain that is worse at night and improves dramatically with aspirin. The characteristic findings for this tumor in clinical and radiologic examinations can, in many instances, lead to a high level of diagnostic confidence. Treatment consists of complete removal of the nidus.

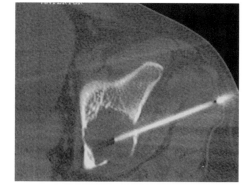

Fig. 4. Radiofrequency ablation. Radiofrequency needle electrode inserted into a destructive iliac lesion.

Conventional treatment is surgical or percutaneous excision. The ability to precisely control the treated area, a high degree of precision, applicability in joints, and excellent dose-response characteristics make interstitial laser photocoagulation a valuable treatment method for osteoid osteoma. The penetration of the needle into the nidus is extremely painful, and the intervention is performed under neuroleptanalgesia or regional block (Fig. 4). General anesthesia is used in children. The hole needed to introduce the fiber is smaller than the other percutaneous ablation techniques. Interstitial laser photocoagulation seems to be a safe and effective way to treat this benign tumor, avoiding the potential complications of the excisional procedure. Surgical treatment of osteoid osteomas should be applied only in inaccessible locations or in tumors localized too near vital structures for percutaneous treatment. In osteoid osteoma, the cure rate with one treatment is 91.6% (77 of 84 patients). The results are similar to radiofrequency ablation in painful bone metastases; however, the ablation size is smaller [11].

Radiofrequency ablation

Radiofrequency ablation is one of the most promising thermal techniques for the treatment of nonresectable tumors. The use of radiofrequency ablation for malignancy was first reported in 1990 for the treatment of hepatic tumors [12]. During radiofrequency ablation, an alternating electric current operated in the range of radio frequency can produce a focal thermal injury in living tissue. Shielded needle electrodes are used to concentrate the energy in selected areas. The tip of the electrode conducts the current, which causes local ionic agitation and subsequent frictional heat, leading to localized coagulation necrosis.

Radiofrequency ablation reduces tumor pain by the physical destruction of sensory nerve fibers in the periosteum and cortex. The decrease in tumor volume following the ablation also reduces the mechanical stimulation of nerve fibers. In addition, radiofrequency ablation destroys tumor cells that produce nerve-stimulating cytokines such as tumor necrosis factor α and various interleukins while inhibiting osteoclast activity [13].

For a complete ablation, the tumor size should be less than 4 cm in diameter. Primary benign tumors like osteoid osteoma can also be successfully treated with radiofrequency ablation.

The best indications for radiofrequency in bone in the authors' opinion are painful bone metastases that cannot be treated by alcohol (ie, risk of intra-articular leak, risk of accidental neurolysis); ablation of large bone metastases of thyroid cancer in association with iodine 131 therapy; and large osteoid osteoma or osteoblastoma.

The length of a single procedure depends on the number of ablations performed. Multiple sessions can be performed. The procedure can be performed under sedation with local or general anesthetic. The choice of guidance system is largely based on operator preference and local experience. Several commercially available generators and electrodes can be used. Grounding electrodes are placed on the patient, and the needle electrode (16–18 G) is inserted into the area to be treated (Fig. 5).

The generator is turned on. Treatment is guided by monitoring temperature or by impedance of the target tissue depending on the type of electrode and generator used (eg, RITA Medical systems, Mountain View, California; Radiotherapeutics Corp., Mountain

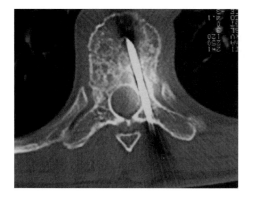

Fig. 5. Vertebroplasty. Transpedicular entry into thoracic vertebrae.

View, California; Radionics, Burlington, Massachusetts; and Berchtold systems, Tuttlingen, Germany).

In metastatic lesions, pain relief is rapidly achieved in 59% of patients at 4 weeks post treatment, with 95% of patients experiencing significant relief at 12 weeks [3]. Rosenthal and colleagues [14] reported on 263 patients who underwent 271 radiofrequency ablation procedures for the removal of an osteoid osteoma over a period of 11 years. The rate of complications was <1%, and successful ablation was achieved in 91% of the patients who had a primary lesion. Of those who had a recurrent osteoid osteoma, 60% were successfully treated with a second radiofrequency ablation procedure.

Adverse effects described are skin burns from the grounding pads, delayed fracture, and transient sphincter dysfunction [3]. Contraindications include lesions close (<1 cm) to vital structures, large lesions (>10 cm), and blastic tumors.

Percutaneous vertebroplasty

Percutaneous vertebroplasty (PVP) is a minimally invasive technique whereby polymethylmethacrylate (bone cement) is injected into a vertebral body. The sole indication for its use is to relieve pain in vertebrae affected by disease (tumor infiltration or vertebral collapse). PVP was originally used to treat the painful aggressive variant of vertebral hemangioma [15] but its use has been extended to painful lesions caused by malignant disease, osteoporotic vertebral wedge fractures, and less common conditions such as Langerhans cell histiocytosis and osteogenesis imperfecta [16].

The precise analgesic mechanism of action PVP is uncertain. The strengthening effect of the cement is thought to stabilize microfractures. The pain-reducing effect of cement cannot be explained by consolidation of the pathologic bone alone. In fact, good pain relief is obtained after injection of only 2 mL of cement in metastasic lesions. Another possible mechanism is that the exothermic effect of the cement polymerization directly damages interosseous or periosteal nerves and directly damages tumor cells. PVP can be performed using fluoroscopy alone or in tandem with CT (the latter being more useful in cervical and transthoracic procedures). The procedure can be performed under sedation or general anesthetic, and a vertebral body biopsy can be performed at the same time.

The route of needle (10–11 G) insertion is dictated by the level to be treated. A transpedicular route is most commonly used (Fig. 6), although anterolateral (cervical), intercostovertebral (thoracic), posterolateral (lumbar), or even a transoral (C2) can be used. A single unipedicular approach is usual, although a bipedicular approach can be employed (the former reducing trauma and procedural time). When the needle is correctly positioned, the bone cement is mixed and injected. At this time, it is vital to watch closely for leakage of cement. When the required amount of cement has been injected, the needle is withdrawn (Fig. 7). Up to three to five levels can be treated in a single session. Patients are able to mobilize within their level of comfort when they have recovered from the anesthetic/sedation.

Using this technique, around 83% of patients who have metastatic disease obtain satisfactory pain relief [17]. Pain relief is not related to the proportion of lesion injected in cases of metastatic disease or myeloma [18].

Complications are low: 6% asymptomatic epidural leak, 1.6% neuralgic pain due to epidural leakage, and 1% asymptomatic pulmonary embolism [17]. Other, rare complications include rib and pedicle fractures, postprocedure deep venous thrombosis, and spinal cord damage. The presence of bone cement does not preclude MRI scans, which can be performed to follow disease progression. Absolute contraindications to this technique include active infection and epidural extension of metastatic tumor with compression of neural structures. Relative contraindications include patients having more than five metastases or diffuse metastases, the presence of radicular pain, fracture of the posterior cortex (increased risk of cement leak), vertebral collapse greater than 70% of body height (needle placement may be difficult), and spinal canal stenosis (asymp-

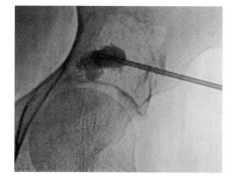

Fig. 7. Osteoplasty. Bone cement injection with filling of an ostoelytic lesion of the superior acetabulum.

tomatic retropulsion of a fracture fragment causing significant spinal canal compromise).

Kyphoplasty

Kyphoplasty combines the techniques of vertebroplasty and angioplasty. The aim of kyphoplasty is pain relief combined with restoration of vertebral body height and reduction in kyphosis. This aim is achieved by "expanding" the fractured vertebra with a balloon and filling the resultant cavity with bone cement. The indications for kyphoplasty are the same as those for vertebroplasty.

Kyphoplasty offers the theoretic advantages of restoration of a degree of vertebral height, reducing deformity, and improving spinal biomechanics. The generation of a cavity within the vertebral body allows low-pressure filling with cement, greatly reducing the risk of cement leakage. Gaitanis and colleagues [19] demonstrated that 96.9% of patients exhibited significant and immediate pain improvement following kyphoplasty. Ninety percent responded within 24 hours. Kyphosis correction was achieved in 89.6%, with a mean correction of 7.6°. Cement leakage occurred in 8.3% of the tumor group but had no clinical consequences.

Osteoplasty

Percutaneous injection of methylmethacrylate (osteoplasty) allows pain reduction and bone strengthening in patients who have malignant pelvic osteolyses who are unable to tolerate surgery. It is most commonly used to improve mobility in patients who have osteolysis involving the weight-bearing part of the acetabulum (ie, the acetabular roof). The proce-

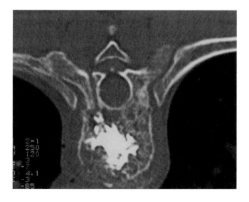

Fig. 6. Vertebroplasty. Postvertebroplasty appearance on CT. Note the dense bone cement in the center of the vertebral body.

dure is similar to that for vertebroplasty. A 10-G needle is positioned within the lesion, and bone cement is injected until the lesion fills or leakage of cement is seen (3.5–11 mL are typically required).

Excellent results can be obtained, with significant pain relief and improved mobility seen in 92% of patients in one series [20]. Contraindications to this technique include local infection and uncorrected coagulopathy. A relative contraindication is the presence of osteolysis of the acetabular fossa, with the risk of traumatic acetabular protrusion on weight bearing. The improved pain relief and mobility afforded by this technique may be detrimental in this group.

The major complication is intra-articular injection in acetabular lesions. This risk is minimized by monitoring the bone filling with fluoroscopic guidance. The next most serious complication is infection; to avoid this complication, strict sterility during the intervention is mandatory.

Arterial intervention

Arterial catheterization has two roles in orthopedic oncology: (1) to allow selective embolization of tumors to reduce their vascularity (ie, preoperatively, for pain relief or to reduce tumor size); and (2) to allow regional infusion of chemotherapeutic agent (ie, in osteosarcoma).

Devascularization of tumors

Arterial embolization has found a role in devascularizing hypervascular tumors before resection. Embolization is particularly important in cases of large tumors that are located in sites in which tourniquet control is not possible. This methodology can also result in decreased intraoperative blood loss, reduced tumor size, and improved visualization of the tumor at surgery. In addition, embolization can be a primary treatment for tumors that are refractory to other forms of treatment (eg, giant cell tumors [21] and aneurysmal bone cysts). Embolization can be used to palliate patients who are poor candidates for surgery.

The goal of embolization is to occlude the blood supply to the tumor without impairing the circulation to surrounding normal tissue. Although most experience of tumor embolization has involved metastatic renal cell carcinomas (70% of which are hypervascular), any hypervascular tumor supplied by large segmental arteries may potentially benefit from embolization (eg, thyroid carcinoma, neuroendocrine

tumors, leiomyosarcomas, and angiosarcomas). Myeloma and melanoma are hypervascular due to a rich capillary network and respond poorly to embolization. Common bone metastasis such as breast, colon, and lung carcinomas are relatively avascular and respond poorly to embolization.

Embolic agents include particles (polyvinyl alcohol particles), liquid (absolute alcohol), or coils. Polyvinyl alcohol particles are most often used and provide permanent occlusion of the target vessel. The size of the polyvinyl alcohol particles is chosen to occlude the capillary bed within the tumor and to be too large to pass through normal vascular anastomosis. Embolization is unsuccessful if the level of occlusion is too proximal. Most embolizations can be completed in a single session, although multiple procedures can be undertaken. If embolization is performed before operative treatment to prevent blood loss, then surgery should be performed within 24 to 48 hours for optimal results [22]. Complete embolization can be achieved in 50% to 86% of patients who have tumors of the spine [22].

Studies have demonstrated a significant reduction in intraoperative blood loss following successful embolization [23,24]. Embolization has the potential to reduce operating time, allow a more extensive resection, and reduce complications in lesions close to important structures such as the spinal cord.

Embolization can be used to palliate symptoms of pain and neural compromise in patients who are unable to tolerate surgical resection. The mechanism of pain relief is uncertain but it may relate to depressurizing the tumor mass, which decreases the pressure on adjacent periosteal nerves. Pain relief occurs at 12 hours to several days following embolization.

Embolization has been used as an alternative to radiotherapy for malignant spinal cord compression. The small amount of cases described in the literature show promising results. O'Reilly and colleagues [25] treated three patients who had acute spinal cord compression from isolated renal cell metastases following failure of radiotherapy and corticosteroids. These patients all improved in terms of pain relief within 24 hours and saw their neurologic function improve. These results lasted longer than 3 to 9 months.

In most studies, serious complication rates are low (1%–2%) following embolization [22]. Serious complications include paraplegia, quadraparesis, and aortic dissection. Forty-three percent of patients experience postembolization syndrome (local pain, low-grade fever, and malaise) following embolization procedures [26].

Direct percutaneous puncture and intralesional injection of the embolic agent can be performed when selective catheterization of a feeding artery is not possible or there is close association between the vascular supply to the tumor and that of important structures such as the spinal cord. Devascularization occurs by occlusion of intratumoral vessels rather than the supplying vessel. This technique has been used successfully in aggressive vertebral body hemangiomas (followed by vertebroplasty).

Embolization has been described as a method for treating giant cell tumors. In one series, sequential embolization resulted in complete relief of pain and radiographic healing in 48% of patients who had giant cell tumors of the axial skeleton [27]. The embolization of sacral giant cell tumors has been described, with some success. Lackman and colleagues [28] described the embolization of 5 sacral giant cell tumors. Four patients gained a complete restoration of function and arrest of tumor growth. Lin and coworkers [22] described embolization of 18 sacral giant cell tumors. In this group of 18 patients, 14 responded favorably to embolization, with improvement in pain and neurologic symptoms. This group also used intra-arterial cisplatin, although it was found that the long-term outcome was not affected by its use. These tumors were those that had not responded to other forms of treatment. Embolization of aneurysmal bone cysts has been performed as a primary treatment. Boriani and colleagues [29] reported on four cases of aneurysmal bone cysts treated with embolization; three were cured by the procedure.

When a single vessel supplies an osteosarcoma, selective catheterization and infusion of chemotherapy is the optimal approach [30]. The rationale for regional chemotherapy is that it maximizes local delivery of the drug, theoretically increasing the local response rate while still allowing a high enough concentration of the drug systemically to affect micrometastases. This regional chemotherapeutic technique facilitates local resection and limb salvage rather than amputation. The administration of chemotherapy (whether it is intra-arterial or intravenous) allows the identification of the best chemotherapy for adjuvant therapy from the degree of necrosis demonstrated in the resected specimen.

The procedure is performed under local anesthetic with or without sedation. Arterial access is usually obtained by puncturing the common femoral artery using a standard Seldinger technique. A 4F catheter is introduced, and the tip is positioned proximal to the hypertrophied vessels that supply the tumor. A catheter with multiple side holes is used to prevent accidental selection of a small side branch vessel with the risk of skin necrosis. The use of this type of catheter produces a degree of turbulent flow to facilitate mixing of the drugs to avoid heterogeneous delivery to the tumor.

Using a combination of intra-arterial cisplatin followed by intravenous doxirubicin, limb salvage surgery is now possible in 80% of patients who have osteosarcoma [31]. Researchers at the M.D. Anderson Cancer Center reviewed 155 intra-arterial infusions of cis-platinum in 42 patients from 1999 to 2002 (unpublished data). The procedure was found to be safe, with no reported instances of skin necrosis, thrombosis, infection, neuropathy, or compartment syndrome. There were seven painful burns (in 6 patients) consisting of skin erythema and induration [29].

Summary

The management of patients who have malignant disorders of bone requires the input of a multidisciplinary team. Most patients are treated with the standard treatments of surgery, radiotherapy, chemotherapy, and hormonal manipulation. If these treatments fail or are contraindicated, then the techniques described in this article may prove beneficial. Minimally invasive techniques used by interventional radiologists can play an important role in reducing pain and improving quality of life for people suffering from these disorders. Accurate localization of treatment areas improves the efficacy of treatment and minimizes potential complications.

References

[1] Shepherd S. Radiotherapy and the management of metastatic bone pain. Clin Radiol 1988;39:547–50.

[2] Gilbert HA, Kagam AR, Nussbaum H, et al. Evaluation of radiation therapy for bone metastases: pain relief and quality of life. AJR Am J Roentgenol 1977; 129:1095–6.

[3] Goetz MP, Callstrom MR, Charboneau JW, et al. Percutaneous image-guided radiofrequency ablation of painful metastases involving bone: a multicenter study. J Clin Oncol 2004;22(2):300–6.

[4] Dupuy DE, Rosenberg AE, Punyaratabandhu T, et al. Accuracy of CT-guided needle biopsy of musculoskeletal neoplasms. AJR Am J Roentgenol 1998; 171(3):759–62.

[5] Murphy WA, Destouet JM, Gilula LA. Percutaneous skeletal biopsy: a procedure for radiologists. Radiology 1981;139:545–9.

[6] Pereira PL, Fritz J, Koenig CW, et al. Preoperative marking of musculoskeletal tumors guided by magnetic resonance imaging. J Bone Joint Surg Am 2004;86(8):1761–7.

[7] Gangi A, Kastler B, Klinkert A, et al. Injection of alcohol into bone metastases under CT guidance. J Comput Assist Tomogr 1994;18(6):932–5.

[8] Gangi A, Dietemann JL, Schultz A, et al. Interventional radiologic procedures with CT guidance in cancer pain management. Radiographics 1996;16: 1289–304.

[9] Campa III JA, Payne R. The management of intractable bone pain: a clinician's perspective. Semin Nucl Med 1992;22(1):3–10.

[10] Gangi A, Dietemann JL, Gasser B, et al. Interventional radiology with laser in bone and joint. Radiol Clin N Am 1998;3:547–59.

[11] Gangi A, Dietemann JL, Gasser B, et al. Percutaneous laser-photocoagulation of osteoid osteomas. Semin Musculoskelet Radiol 1997;1(2):273–80.

[12] McGahan JP, Browning PD, Brock JM, et al. Hepatic ablation using radiofrequency electrocautery. Invest Radiol 1990;25:267–70.

[13] Callstrom MR, Charboneau JW, Goetz MP, et al. Painful metastases involving bone: feasibility of percutaneous CT- and US-guided radio-frequency ablation. Radiology 2002;224:87–97.

[14] Rosenthal DI, Hornicek FJ, Torriani M, et al. Osteoid osteoma: percutaneous treatment with radiofrequency energy. Radiology 2003;229:171–5.

[15] Galibert P, Deramond H, Rosat P, et al. Preliminary note on the treatment of vertebral angioma by percutaneous acrylic vertebroplasty. Neurochirurgie 1987; 33:166–8.

[16] Rami PM, McGraw JK, Heatwole EV, et al. Percutaneous vertebroplasty in the treatment of vertebral body compression fracture secondary to osteogenesis imperfecta [Epub Dec 18, 2001; erratum in Skeletal Radiol 2002;31(9):558]. Skeletal Radiol 2002;31(3): 162–5.

[17] Gangi A, Dietemann JL, Guth S, et al. Computed tomography (CT) and fluoroscopy-guided vertebroplasty: results and complications in 187 patients. Semin Intervent Radiol 1999;200:525–30.

[18] Cotten A, Dewatre F, Cortet B, et al. Percutaneous vertebroplasty for osteolytic metastases and myeloma: effects of the percentage of lesion filling and the leakage of methyl methacrylate at clinical follow-up. Radiology 1996;200(2):525–30.

[19] Gaitanis IN, Hadjipavlou AG, Katonis PG, et al. Balloon kyphoplasty for the treatment of pathological vertebral compressive fractures [Epub Oct 8, 2004]. Eur Spine J 2005;14(3):250–60.

[20] Kelekis A, Lovblad KO, Mehdizade A, et al. Pelvic osteoplasty in osteolytic metastases: technical approach under fluoroscopic guidance and early clinical results. J Vasc Interv Radiol 2005;16(1):81–8.

[21] Lin PP, Guzel VB, Moura MF, et al. Long-term follow-up of patients with giant cell tumor of the sacrum treated with selective arterial embolization. Cancer 2002;95(6):1317–25.

[22] Gottfried ON, Schloesser PE, Schmidt MH, et al. Embolization of metastatic spinal tumors. Neurosurg Clin N Am 2004;15(4):391–9.

[23] Sun S, Lang EV. Bone metastases from renal cell carcinoma: preoperative embolization. J Vasc Interv Radiol 1998;9:263–9.

[24] Manke C, Bretschneider T, Lenhart M, et al. Spinal metastases from renal cell carcinoma: effect of preoperative particle embolization on intraoperative blood loss. AJNR Am J Neuroradiol 2001;22(5):997–1003.

[25] O'Reilly GV, Kleefield J, Klein LA, et al. Embolization of solitary spinal metastases from renal cell carcinoma: alternative therapy for spinal cord or nerve root compression. Surg Neurol 1989;31(4):268–71.

[26] Hemingway AP, Allison DJ. Complications of embolization: analysis of 410 procedures. Radiology 1988;166(3):669–72.

[27] Carrasco CH. Radiological management of bone tumours. In: Dondelinger RF, Kurdziel JC, Rossi P, et al, editors. Interventional radiology. Stuttgart, Germany: Thieme; 1990. p. 489–97.

[28] Lackman RD, Khoury LD, Esmail A, et al. The treatment of sacral giant-cell tumours by serial arterial embolisation. J Bone Joint Surg Br 2002;84(6):873–7.

[29] Boriani S, DeIure F, Campanacci L, et al. Aneurysmal bone cyst of the mobile spine: report on 41 cases. Spine 2001;26(1):27–35.

[30] Wallace MJ, Wallace S. Chemoembolization, infusion and embolization. In: Adam A, Dondelinger RF, Mueller PR, editors. Interventional radiology in cancer. Berlin: Springer–Verlag; 2004. p. 179–224.

[31] Weber KL. What's new in musculoskeletal oncology. J Bone Joint Surg Am 2004;86(5):1104–9.

ELSEVIER
SAUNDERS

Orthop Clin N Am 37 (2006) 113–117

ORTHOPEDIC
CLINICS
OF NORTH AMERICA

Index

Note: Page numbers of article titles are in **boldface** type.

0030-5898/06/$ – see front matter © 2005 Elsevier Inc. All rights reserved.
doi:10.1016/S0030-5898(05)00112-4

orthopedic.theclinics.com

Changing Your Address?

Make sure your subscription changes too! When you notify us of your new address, you can help make our job easier by including an exact copy of your Clinics label number with your old address (see illustration below.) This number identifies you to our computer system and will speed the processing of your address change. Please be sure this label number accompanies your old address and your corrected address—you can send an old Clinics label with your number on it or just copy it exactly and send it to the address listed below.

We appreciate your help in our attempt to give you continuous coverage. Thank you.

W. B. Saunders Company

SHIPPING AND RECEIVING DEPTS.
151 BENIGNO BLVD.
BELLMAWR, N.J. 08031

SECOND CLASS POSTAGE
PAID AT BELLMAWR, N.J.

This is your copy of the
_____ **CLINICS OF NORTH AMERICA**

00503570 DOE—J32400   101   NH   8102

JOHN C DOE MD
324 SAMSON ST
BERLIN   NH   03570

XP-D11494

JAN ISSUE

Your Clinics Label Number

Copy it exactly or send your label
along with your address to:
W.B. Saunders Company, Customer Service
Orlando, FL 32887-4800
Call Toll Free 1-800-654-2452

Please allow four to six weeks for delivery of new subscriptions and for processing address changes.